THE BODYBUILDER

8 SIMPLE STEPS TO ACHIEVE
PHYSICAL AND SPIRITUAL GROWTH

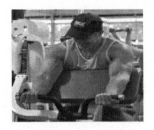

ANTHONY L. PELELLA

WWW.THEBODYBUILDERBOOK.COM

ISBN-13:978-0692413982 (sc)
ISBN-10:0692413987

Library of Congress Control Number: 2013902920

Printed in the United States of America

This book is printed on acid-free paper.

FOR <u>PHYSICAL TRAINING</u> IS OF **SOME**
VALUE, BUT <u>GODLINESS</u> HAS VALUE FOR
ALL THINGS, HOLDING PROMISE FOR BOTH
THE PRESENT LIFE AND THE LIFE TO COME.
—1 TIMOTHY 4:8

WWW.THEBODYBUILDERBOOK.COM

CONTENTS

Preface: What Is This All About?   xi

Chapter 1: I Can't Get No Satisfaction   1

Chapter 2: You Know, I Used to Look Like That!   11

Chapter 3: You Are What You Eat   27

Chapter 4: The Training Partner   43

Chapter 5: A Firm Foundation   55

Chapter 6: Sacrifice   69

Chapter 7: A "Rested" Development   87

Chapter 8: The Change-Up   99

Conclusion: The Spirit of the Radio   113

WWW.THEBODYBUILDERBOOK.COM

DEDICATION

In this life I have received many great gifts from the Lord. First is my salvation through Jesus Christ. In 1995 I received the gift of my wife DyAnna. In 2002 & 2004 it was the gifts of my daughters Gianna & Alyssa. They have all brought me so much joy and have made my world what it is today. We serve God together, live life together & are a true family. They all have created an atmosphere in my life to be able to write about the things that I do. DyAnna, thank you for being my biggest fan during this process. Girls, thank you for all the love you give daddy and all the time you are willing to give me up so I can help others. I also want to thank my dad. He instilled in me at an early age the desire to train and the desire to love Jesus with all my heart.

PREFACE: WHAT IS THIS ALL ABOUT?

Physical Training:

It was fall 1990 when my dream came true and I stepped on stage for the first time. The announcing of my name, the shouts of the crowd, the bright lights, the booming music—looking back, it seems like just a blur, but it was really me, and I deserved to be up there. For ninety seconds, the stage belonged to me, and I held my own against some stiff competition. Although I didn't place in the top five of my weight class, I placed in the eyes of my dad, which really meant more to me than a trophy.

Coming from a home where my dad was a dedicated weightlifter truly shaped my life from a young age. Over the years, when my friends would ask my dad to "make a muscle," I felt great pride. The kids would sit on the seats of their Huffy bikes at the end of the driveway and watch as my dad, and sometimes his friends, would lift massive weights. We would all watch and wish that one day we could look like them! Growing up in Brentwood during the '70s, I watched my dad train. In Valley Stream during the '80s, I started training with him. It was during these training sessions that I gleaned many of these valuable lessons you will read about.

For several years I pushed myself to be the best-built guy I could be, but it wasn't until 1990 when it all came together. My father introduced me to his friend Marshall Gough, who also happened to be the current Mr. Sanitation NYC. Marshall started training me and invited me to see him compete in the city. Eventually we agreed that I would get ready for my first show, which led to another important meeting for me. Marshall introduced me to Mr. Charlie Carollo, owner of Fifth Avenue Gym in Brooklyn, which was pumping out some of the best competitors on the East Coast at the time. After my thorough evaluation by both Charlie and Marshall, it was time to go to work. *No longer was I going to be another guy who worked out; I was going to be a bodybuilder.*

Eventually I entered an NPC show called the Natural New York City, which was the show I mentioned earlier. This show got me hungry and caused me to want more. I entered two more shows in the next two years and set my eyes on some big dreams of what I might one day become. I had won several trophies and even had my name and some good reviews in *Natural Physique Magazine.* Yet nothing was as rewarding and fulfilling as the "phone call." My dad had called the day after my first show and told me of how proud he was. He said he would never have had the nerve to go up there on that stage and do what I did, and in some way he was living a dream through me. He was proud, and he made sure he told me! I had the approval of my father, and honestly, that was the greatest reward of all.

Godliness:

It was 1991, and I was pretty down on life. It was in my family's best interest for me to move out of the house. Shortly after that I had my car repossessed, and then my girlfriend of three years broke up with me. It kind of all came down heavy when I realized I didn't even have enough money to buy the asthma medicine I needed just to catch my breath. Again, to say I was down on life is a pretty subtle way to describe how I was feeling.

For a large part of my upbringing, God was taught but not necessarily lived. What I mean is that I had religion classes as a kid, was brought to Sunday school as I grew up, and sat in services like a good boy. Well, I should say sometimes, and many times reluctantly at that. Life itself was never bad, but God was never a true priority for me. I might have cried at times when I heard a great sermon about Jesus. I did some nice things because I felt that's what God would want, but I never really lived for Jesus. He would only get my leftovers.

As I got older, other things became my priorities, like partying with friends, getting popular, driving a cool car (not to mention all the bombs I drove before I got my '70 Chevelle), and chasing after girls. God was a thought but not a conviction. I would always hope the preacher would get done quickly so I wouldn't miss kickoff. I loved the 4:00 p.m. kickoffs. I never had to miss a second. Remember, this was before the DVR generation, and I'm a huge Giants fan. My mind was clouded with a lot of things, most of which had no concern about heaven or hell, Jesus or Satan, or whether I was saved or a sinner.

I remember going to my dad's house just after my girlfriend and I broke up. I was pretty much a mess. He felt really bad and gave me the first part of his somewhat truthful advice. He said, "Son, just keep working out. The irons will never let you down." Not exactly what you want to hear when you're hurting over a girlfriend, but that's Dad. He didn't stop there though. He shortly after had me meet with my pastor. We hung out together in my basement apartment, and we all had a heart-to-heart talk. That night I truly realized what needed to be done. I needed to ask Jesus to forgive me of my sins and surrender my life to Him. That's just what I did. I believe that night was the start of something great.

Why would I say the start? Because on that night I chose to move away from my church and Christian friends and live in Michigan with my mom. There I got caught up in all the nonsense I was doing back in Long Island. It was no fault of my mom's. I was too old to be told what to do. Eventually I found my way back home, only to be the same Anthony again. I would say about a few months after moving back, "It happened." What, you ask? I'll tell you. I was in front of my house in Valley Stream talking to my dad about what I was up to when he asked me, "Son, when are you going to get your life right with Jesus?" I'm telling you, the clouds opened for me. Just by hearing those words, I made a choice that finally backed up that decision I had made in my basement several months earlier.

Man, it was like I walked through a doorway. All of the sudden, the birds chirped different, the trees swayed different, and even the breeze felt different. I knew in my heart I was going to be committed to the ways of God's Word for the rest of my life. *No longer would I just be another kid who went to church; I was going to be a follower of Jesus.* There are many wonderful things that have happened to me during this awesome journey I call my Christian walk. Yet none of these things comes close to equaling the thought of knowing I have the approval of my heavenly Father, and honestly, that's the greatest reward of all.

This book is a series of chapters that will show the amazing parallels between two of my greatest passions in life prior to getting married and having children: Jesus and bodybuilding. Now it's Jesus and my family. The church is third, and physical training comes in somewhere close to that.

Each chapter will contain what I believe to be amazing parallels between the human body and the body of Christ.

1) The way God has developed the human body to grow as a result of several different challenges.

2) The way God has developed the church (His body) to grow as a result of several different challenges.

Oh, by the way, for the rest of this book I will be referring to the church as "the body" because that is the term used by the Bible so often to describe all those who know Christ as Lord and Savior. To validate my ability to write in these areas with confidence, let me give you my background:

In the physical training area, I not only was a novice bodybuilding competitor, but I also have twenty-seven years of hands-on training experience. I was also a certified personal trainer with AFFA from1999 to 2001.

In the area of godliness, I have been living for Christ faithfully for twenty-two years. I have a one-year certificate of study from Zion Bible College. I am currently an Assemblies of God–ordained minister in the New York district and have been senior pastor of Medford Assembly of God for close to twenty years.

Each chapter will be broken down in two main sections, as you have read in my opening comments. The "Physical Training" sections explain the work we put into building a healthy and great body. The "Godliness" sections explain the work God does in us to build a healthy and great body.

No matter how you look at it, Jesus is:

"THE BODY BUILDER".

WWW.THEBODYBUILDERBOOK.COM

CHAPTER 1

I CAN'T GET NO SATISFACTION

I'm not satisfied, I want more weight. I want to beat him.
—Lou Ferrigno, *Pumping Iron*

Blessed are those who hunger and thirst for righteousness, for they will be filled. (Matt. 5:6)

Physical Training:

Let me draw you the scene. I'm a little kid hanging out with my dad, watching this movie he couldn't wait to see. It was called *Pumping Iron*. This was one of the first movies ever on the life and rituals of hardcore bodybuilders. It follows Arnold, Franco, Louie, and so on. Although it really showcased the greatest bodybuilder of all time, Arnold Schwarzenegger, my attention was drawn to my favorite superhero, Lou Ferrigno. I'll never forget watching Louie and his dad going into the gym and training for the big show against Arnold. And then, the moment that gives me chills to this day took place. As Lou was lifting a ton of weight over his head, he slammed the weight on the rack. With passion, anger, and an incredibly competitive spirit, he yelled, "I'm not satisfied. I want more weight. I want to beat him."

Wow! When most people would have said enough, Louie said more. As a kid, that line moved me. It motivated me, and I have to tell you, it still does today. The reason it made such an impact on me is that I lived with that passion in me for so long. In fact, I still do. I knew when I began to train at about fifteen years old that there was something more for me. I wasn't meant to be a lean kid who was pretty athletic. I was not satisfied with how I looked or what I could lift. I had gotten the bug. Whatever it was going to take, I was going to do it. I didn't want to just be a guy who looked like he worked out; I wanted to be the best-built guy in school, the best-built guy in town!

I realized I was missing something in my life, and now I had found it. I tried baseball and football. I really loved playing them both. I tried hockey, but if you can't skate, you're done. There was nothing like the gym—nothing like the pump. There was nothing like the looks you got from guys who were in awe and girls who—well, let's leave it at that.

Face it—you have to be a little egotistical to be a bodybuilder. You're always checking yourself out and looking in a mirror to see how good you look. Sounds like vanity, I know. Yet it wasn't the way many committed lifters thought of it. You were in a different place.

When you flexed in the mirror, you weren't saying, "I'm better than you"; you were saying, "Am I getting the results I'm striving for? Am I making good gains? Where do I need to improve? What are my weak points?" As Arnold described it in *Pumping Iron,* you are like a lump of clay, and training helps you sculpt the body you are trying to achieve.

Nothing got my attention more than training. My mind was always thinking about it. My mouth was always talking about it. My clothes were always propagating it. (That's because I always wore my shirts a size too small.) I had found my calling. I was finally figuring out who I was going to be: a bodybuilder. I had to sleep, eat, drink, and breathe it all day long. This brings me to my next point.

When you start out lifting to truly change your body, you realize just how unsatisfied you really are with how you look. You realize this is going to be a marathon, not a sprint. At the end of the day, if you are not in contest shape, there is no one to blame but yourself. There is no team to point fingers at, no coach to stand in your place on the stage. You alone are either blamed or applauded. Either way, it's up to you, and when you realize the judges won't go easy on you simply because you're nice, you won't accept the easy road.

Not being satisfied with where I was and knowing that strict judging was coming my way pushed me to heights I never dreamed of. Like Big Louie, I knew what it meant to desire to always beat my personal best. If I benched 350, I wanted 375. If I squatted 500, I wanted 525. I always wanted to go further than I could have imagined. I always wanted to challenge myself to improve. When you're satisfied with how you look, you get complacent. You tend to slack on diet and training. Trust me—I have done both and regretted it. When you do this, you look back at the time you wasted and wish you had used it wisely and trained instead of playing games.

I would always ask myself, "What would I look like now if I hadn't skipped my diet for the last two months?" Or "What would I look like now if I had kept training as hard as I did last year?" The shoulda, woulda, coulda blues. Man, I wish I could get back some of that wasted time and use it to bring out the potential I know is locked away in me.

Basically, it came down to this for me: There were several things in life that made me happy. Bodybuilding was different. Bodybuilding gave me joy! It satisfied me. I felt incomplete unless I was in the gym. I felt lost if I cheated on my diet. If you looked at Anthony Pelella, you knew he lifted. If you talked to him, you knew he lifted. Bodybuilding was evident in my physical appearance and in my heart. This might sound strange, but try to follow me. I would never be satisfied with my appearance because I knew I could always get better, yet I was finally satisfied because I knew who I was going to become!

Godliness:

It is amazing to me how long I ran away from God. I tried to serve Him on my terms, justifying my sinful ways with petty excuses that would never cut it in heaven. All the while, I never truly felt satisfied. I always had this empty feeling i n s i d e.

Now don't get me wrong—I had my share of fun, as many of you reading this may understand. I always had a girl to hang out with. Being both a weightlifter and not too ugly helped. I had a cool group of friends who really had a lot of fun. I made decent money at the construction business I worked for. I was even working at night in one of the most popular night clubs on Long Island, called Malibu. It was huge and had two different sides to it. One side was a disco; the other was new wave. That's what they called it in the eighties.

I was a bar back and served drinks at parties. I got pretty cool favors during club nights since I knew the staff. I had access to the private Malibu beach club, which was impressive to ladies. Finally, I was making strides to possibly get that bouncing job I wanted. This would seal the deal. Everyone loves the bouncers. I was training hard, looking big, and thinking I could take on anyone. I was pretty content with how things were going.

Even so, something was missing. Despite all this cool stuff happening in my life, I was sure I was missing the mark of what I was here for. I was starting to tear myself in two. To be honest, I was living as a hypocrite. At the same time I was working at the club and engaging in what the Bible would describe as sinful activity, I was working with the kids at my church. I was supposed to be an example for them to look up to and be able to follow Jesus. I knew something wasn't right there. If I was so happy with the club scene and doing life on my terms, why was I getting torn up inside over what I was choosing to do? Then I figured it out. It was because what I was truly looking for was not in the club, with the girls, in a bottle, or as a bouncer. I was looking to have true joy, not to just be happy.

The things that made me happy were temporary. You get a

quick fix, and then you have to run after one again. After the buzz or the high wore off, where did it leave me? Wondering how I could get that feeling again and how long it would take for it to happen. I remembered what Jesus said in His Word, and it started to make sense.

> *Blessed are those who hunger and thirst for righteousness, for they will be filled. (Matt. 5:6)*

If I was to truly be filled with joy, then I needed to be satisfied not by the things I thought were making me happy but with the things that made God happy. Who better to fill me up with exactly what I needed than the one who created me? I also remembered another important passage of the Bible.

> *But seek first his kingdom and his righteousness, and all these things will be given to you as well. (Matt. 6:33)*

I never felt better than when I put this passage to the test. I decided, as I already described to you, to make that decision to give Jesus my all, the way He gave His all for me. I would live for Him and become His servant. I ate, drank, thought, spoke, and breathed the ways of the Lord. I trained myself in the ways of righteousness for His glory and found myself never satisfied with where I was as a Christian.

Today, if I know some Scripture, I want to know more. If I tell someone about Jesus' love, I want to tell more. If I can give some money to help build His church, I want to give more. Now I don't just go to church; I'm a servant in God's house. Now I don't just say a prayer; I seek God's will for my life and spend quality time talking with Him. Amazingly enough, as I lived for Him, He kept His promise. I was, for the first time, truly satisfied in my spirit. I knew who I was supposed to be and was excited about what I could eventually do for His kingdom.

Just like bodybuilding, when I gazed into my life, I realized

God had a lot of work to do in me, and I would never again be satisfied with where I was as a person. I recognized that if I was going to truly stay satisfied, then I was never going to be able to become complacent, accept the status quo, or compromise. Also, like bodybuilding, I realized there would be no one in this world to blame for me slacking off but me. It was my life to live, my choices to make. I would never blame a friend, spouse, pastor, or anyone else for mistakes I might choose to make. There is no finger pointing in Christianity. As it says:

Man is destined to die once, and after that to face judgment. (Heb. 9:27)

We must all give an account for what we do in this world before the Lord Jesus Christ. This account of what I've chosen to do falls on me, and I will do all I can to be sure the God who saved me from my sin will be satisfied with who I have become as a result of what He has been able to do in me. It kind of boils down to what John the Baptist said about Jesus:

He must become greater; I must become less. (John 3:30)

Consider this point also:

Then I saw a great white throne and him who was seated on it. Earth and sky fled from his presence, and there was no place for them. And I saw the dead, great and small, standing before the throne, and books were opened. Another book was opened, which is the book of life. The dead were judged according to what they had done as recorded in the books. (Rev. 20:11–12)

I often thought about how those judges at my shows critiqued my physique. They went over every area of my body to determine if

I was what they were looking for. If I had a weak point (calves!), they would expose it. If I had a good point (biceps), they would applaud it. Nothing got past the judges, and truly, if you weren't really ready to be up on that stage, it was going to be embarrassing.

What about the judge of our souls? What about the God who knows all, is everywhere, and is all powerful? Who among us can escape His view? Who in this world thinks he or she can hide from God the flaws of his or her life—the sins locked away in the past memories of time, the skeletons of shame that no one has been told of. We will all give an account of what we have done, and friends, when we stand on that stage of judgment for our souls, there are one of two things that the wisest judge of all will say.

> *Then I will tell them plainly, "I never knew you. Away from me, you evildoers!" (Matt. 7:23)*

> *Well done, good and faithful servant! You have been faithful with a few things; I will put you in charge of many things. Come and share your master's happiness! (Matt. 25:21)*

Which one you get to hear depends on what you consider to be true satisfaction. I have truly lived life on both sides of the fence. I have lived in a rebellious way and dishonored God with my actions. I have also lived in obedience to Jesus' commands and given my all for Him. There is no contest. The only way to truly find satisfaction and to live with joy that never grows old is to surrender your life to Christ.

Things to Ponder

1) Who are you living for? Who are you living to get approval from? Whose validation of what you do would make you feel like you have arrived?

2) What are you passionate about; what makes you go the extra mile?

3) What is your definition of satisfaction? Does this definition line up with God's?

4) What are some of your weak points in life? Where do you need to improve with God?

5) Can you differentiate between being happy and having joy?

CHAPTER 2

YOU KNOW, I USED TO LOOK LIKE THAT!

—Joe Public

He who overcomes will, like them, be dressed in white. (Rev. 3:20)

Physical Training:

I have found that an amazing thing happens when people identify the goal that you have been shooting for. My goal obviously was to be very muscular and lean and have loads of definition. Even though today I do not dare call myself a bodybuilder, I still train hard and enjoy trying to obtain personally set g o a l s .

It's safe to say there is a remnant of my serious training seen by people who notice my arms, back, or chest. In those moments when someone says, "Hey, do you work out?" a smile creeps in on my face, and I'll generally answer something like, "Yeah, I like to lift some weights." Then the amazing thing takes place. This next sentence is shocking and not for the weak. You may want to sit before reading this next line. Many times those who have made note of my personal gains in muscular fitness say something kind of like this, "You know, I used to look like that when I was working out." I know, it's hard to believe. However, I do need to explain the magnitude of this comment for those who may read this and say, "What's the big deal?"

When I was younger, that comment would get my dander up. Today I just smile and say, "Great, I'm sure you looked really good." Please understand why that comment causes all types of athletes to cringe and leaves a feeling of disrespect to those who have worked so hard to attain the level of excellence they are or were at. Now please, know my heart about this. I'm not mad, upset, or offended by a comment like that. This is, again, not an ego thing. I'm just explaining a truth many people who have dedicated themselves to go above the average person and achieve goals that seem unattainable can relate to.

When a person would tell me they used to look like me, even though they didn't realize it, it was an insult. They were telling me that the milestones I reached, which took years, months, and countless hours dedicated to my sport, they achieved during the few weeks of their health kick back in the day. Most likely the person was training with a Joe Weider sand set and stuck to bench presses and curls because they really didn't know how to work out. In the chapters to come, you will read about the sacrifices made and the discipline required to get the results I did. Honestly, I think it's great that anyone does some type of athletic training, be it weights or sports. It's when I'm told their regimen, which was probably average at best, was equal to my gut-wrenching way of life that I have to disagree.

Sometimes people who make the comment will get validation from their girlfriends or spouses about how they looked. The spouses agree, as they should. They would be asking for trouble if they didn't. Forgive me, I mean no disrespect here, but that spouse is no bodybuilding judge. In my first show, I had Bernard Sealy on my judging panel. He was a former Mr. Olympia competitor. For those of you who don't know, Mr. Olympia is the highest level of competition in the bodybuilding world. Seated with him were other experts in the field of bodybuilding who tore apart every aspect of my physique to be sure I was judged properly. Can you understand why I would be taken back by a judgment call of spouses on how good a loved one looked when he or she did a few reps before bed in high school?

This comment is the same type of statement you hear guys or their parents make about their sons. It goes something like this: "Joey was really a great baseball player. If he would have tried, he probably would have been a pro." Now I have a pro golfer in our church whose name is Paul. He is the Head Golf Pro at an exclusive Country Club located here on Long Island. Paul is awesome at his field of expertise. Often we read about him playing in high-pressure tournaments all over the New York area. In fact, not very long ago, he missed the US Open by one stroke. His caliber of play is well above all the other people I know who have ever played golf. Does anyone have any idea how long it took this man to be able to play on the level he does? Do they know how hard it is to be consistent year after year and to play despite injury and personal situations, and on top of that, to be a dad and h u s b a n d ?

You don't get a pass at his level. Whatever you have to do to keep your game at its peak, you have to do it. On occasion, someone may shoot a round comparable to him or maybe even beat him by a stroke. Right away their juices start to flow, and they start having visions of grandeur. "Hey, I can do your job. I'm as good as you." Those people have never played with the pressure this man has to face. *Everyone likes to yell at the batter who strikes out looking as if they could have hit the ball over the wall. It's so easy to be a Monday-morning quarterback, especially when you don't have crazy linebackers trying to tear your head off!* The practice and effort it takes to play at a professional level in golf is mind boggling. Yet there are still those who would say, "I could play like that if I really wanted to." Please remember that thousands of people have wanted to and tried. They dedicated their lives to becoming pros and never were able to cut the mustard.

That's one of the reasons why I do not have a problem with baseball players' salaries. I know they are off the charts and school teachers are underpaid in many cases. I'm not trying to compare the two, but I do know one thing: there are thousands and thousands of teachers doing a great job and worth probably more than they are getting paid. With that said, please listen to the odds of making it into any professional-level sport according to an article written by Walter Leavy in *Ebony* magazine:

> Art Young, director of Urban Youth Sports at Northeastern University's Center for the Study of Sports in Society, came up with some staggering figures concerning the possibility of realizing a dream to become a pro athlete. Based on some extensive studies, he says that only 1 out of every 50,000 high school athletes will ever become a part of a professional team. To put those astronomical odds in perspective, that's like filling each seat at Denver's Coors Field (the home of the Colorado Rockies), then placing each name in a huge barrel. If yours isn't the one, single name drawn, then—just like that—your lifelong dream is dead![1]

1   Walter Leavy, "The Dream to Be like Mike and the Odds of Achieving It," *Ebony Magazine*, November 1998, 34.

Many years ago, I was with a friend of mine on a kind of double-date at Shea Stadium. He was with his soon-to-be wife, and I was with a young lady who wished she was not there. Anyway, they had this moment between innings where they would call a section and seat number out for a chance to win tickets to another game. Would you believe that they called my seat? In fact, the guy who got us the tickets ran down to collect our prize, and they had his picture up on Diamond Vision during the inning after we won. Now think about that. There were about fifty-five thousand seats in Shea. Out of all those cheering fans, I was the one to be declared the winner. The chances of that happening again in my lifetime at any stadium are probably zero. Think about the scene Walter Leavy drew for us. A stadium filled with fifty thousand people, and only one makes it to the top. It's staggering to say the least, and it should remind us of the amazing price that would have to be paid to make this dream a reality.

Do you know how many baseball players there are in the world? There are approximately eleven hundred professional baseball players on the earth. They are a rare breed. Not everyone who seems to be good in high school or at the college level makes it to the pros. It is one of the most difficult positions to hold in the professional work force. The same goes for basketball, football, hockey, boxing, and all other organized and professionally sanctioned sports. To simply state that you could have been a pro but had other things to do is kind of an insult to those who have broken their backs, given their blood, and sacrificed so much to attain that which very few can take hold of.

Godliness:

In my life as a Christian, one of the saddest things I encounter are people who believe that what they did as a child or when they were young was enough to get them into the kingdom of God. Please let me explain what I mean by this. In order to enter heaven, a person must be born again. Now just what does born again mean? In the Bible, Jesus makes a clear statement to a man who was a priest and was supposed to be a teacher of God's Word to the people. This man was asking Jesus what he needed to do to get into heaven. Jesus said:

> *In reply Jesus declared, "I tell you the truth, no one can see the kingdom of God unless he is born again." (John 3:3)*

Jesus didn't want him to join a group or wear a special jacket with the words "born again" on it. He was simply saying you need to truly believe in your heart that Jesus is who He said He was. A passage that followed was able to sum it all u p :

> *For God so loved the world that he gave his one and only Son, that whoever believes in him shall not perish but have eternal life. (John 3:16)*

Those who would come to understand this truth and wanted to receive Christ as Savior were exhorted by the apostle Paul to make a personal confession of their faith to the Lord H i m s e l f .

> *That if you confess with your mouth, "Jesus is Lord," and believe in your heart that God raised him from the dead, you will be saved. (Rom. 10:9)*

With that said, being born again is a point in our lives where we recognize our need as sinners for a Savior. We believe Jesus is that Savior, and it's only through Him that we can find our names written in the Book of Life. Being born again is a condition of one's heart. Remember, salvation is not something we can earn; rather, it is something God has earned for us. We cannot save ourselves from the effects of sin, thus our need to be s a v e d .

Now let me try to explain why I feel so upset about the many people who think they are okay with God even though they live a life very far from the teachings of Jesus. True Christian living is something that has to be worked at and learned as we go. It is not a burden to live for the Lord, but not every moment will be easy. The Bible tells us we need to get into some serious training when it comes to living for Jesus.

> *Have nothing to do with godless myths and old wives' tales; rather, train yourself to be godly. (1 Tim. 4:7)*

Listen to these powerful words written by P a u l :

> *Therefore I do not run like a man running aimlessly; I do not fight like a man beating the air. No, I beat my body and make it my slave so that after I have preached to others, I myself will not be disqualified for the prize. (1 Cor. 9:26–27)*

For some reason, many people have fallen into two traps. One trap is that they go through some basic motions that look godly so when they stand in judgment, they can pull out some type of fire insurance policy that will give God no choice but to accept them. The other is that when they were younger, they did all the right religious things and therefore will be fine when they stand in judgment before God. Unfortunately, both of them are saying the same thing: "I did the religion thing in my life already, so I'll be fine in God's eyes." They are saying, "I used to look like you when it came to God, but now I have other things to do." As insulting as it was to me when someone said they looked like I did physically, imagine how hurtful it is to God when someone tells Him they

17

don't have time for Him, yet He'll have to accept them into His kingdom.

Let's look at the first trap—people who do the bare-bones minimum and hope it will cut the mustard in the eyes of God. One of the things I find American Christians doing very often is what the Bible says:

> **They claim to know God, but by their actions they deny him. (Titus 1:16)**

> **But mark this: There will be terrible times in the last days. People will be lovers of themselves, lovers of money, boastful, proud, abusive, disobedient to their parents, ungrateful, unholy, without love, unforgiving, slanderous, without self-control, brutal, not lovers of the good, treacherous, rash, conceited, lovers of pleasure rather than lovers of God—having a form of godliness but denying its power. (2 Tim. 3:1–5a)**

In other words, at times they look like Christians, they talk like Christians, and they act like Christians, but when a test or temptation comes, they look nothing like Christians. As much as it is important for us to understand that we cannot earn salvation, we need to understand that a life of obedience always follows a true confession of our need for the Savior. A person who acts like a Christian is simply that—an actor. These people put on a mask and play a role for those who may or may not know any better. They feel they will go to church "when they can," practice good morals and ethics, and try to be kind when it is not infringing on their personal rights.

We have not ever been called to act like followers of Jesus; we have been commissioned to "live a life that is worthy of the Lord." Paul the apostle said, "Follow me as I follow Christ." The disciples didn't start out strong and then just do what they wanted because they had arrived. They gave their lives for the cause of spreading the gospel message. That means their everyday living and their actual heart-pumping lives. They lived and died for the cause Jesus birthed in their hearts.

To simply go through a series of rituals and believe that the God of our souls will be pleased is as erroneous as believing you could have been a professional athlete if you felt like it. The comment makes no sense. As my own pastor told me on that day in my basement in 1991, there are no fire insurance policies handed out by the Holy Spirit to those who want to live life on their terms. You cannot be a part-time servant of the Lord. Either you are for Him or against Him. Either you are His child or His enemy.

Think about what happened between Jesus and the rich man:

> *A certain ruler asked him, "Good teacher, what must I do to inherit eternal life?" "Why do you call me good?" Jesus answered. "No one is good-- except God alone. You know the commandments: 'Do not commit adultery, do not murder, do not steal, do not give false testimony, honor your father and mother.'" "All these I have kept since I was a boy," he said. When Jesus heard this, he said to him, "You still lack one thing. Sell everything you have and give to the poor, and you will have treasure in heaven. Then come, follow me." When he heard this, he became very sad, because he was a man of great wealth. Jesus looked at him and said, "How hard it is for the rich to enter the kingdom of God!" (Luke 18:18–24)*

Here we see a man who was good at going through the motions. He did some things he learned growing up and thought maybe that would be enough to carry him through to eternal life. Instead Jesus got to the heart of the matter. In fact, he hit the rich man in the heart by hitting him in the wallet. First Jesus said, "Sell everything you have," and then He said, "Follow me."

First off, the guy did not want to part with his material

possessions, so that meant money was more important than Jesus. Second, Jesus wanted his full attention and have the rich man follow Him. Jesus knew the money issue, unless removed, would keep this guy from getting to where Jesus wants all of us to be—a true follower of the Lord. It may be money or it may be lust or it may be an addiction that's getting in the way. If we do not let the Holy Spirit continue to mold us every day, we are going to miss the kingdom and walk away sad. Don't forget, this rich man had knowledge of what was right and did some of it, but before Jesus asks for our obedience, He wants our hearts. It is just as He said to the Pharisees:

> *Woe to you, teachers of the law and Pharisees, you hypocrites! You give a tenth of your spices—mint, dill and cumin. But you have neglected the more important matters of the law—justice, mercy and faithfulness. You should have practiced the latter, without neglecting the former. (Matt. 23:23)*

Our responsibility is to do just as the Bible says:

> *Find out what pleases the Lord. (Eph. 5:10)*

We also need to realize this simple biblical truth:

> *Then he said to them all: "If anyone would come after me, he must deny himself and take up his cross daily and follow me." (Luke 9:23)*

I was recently talking with Omar Salas of the Latin band El Trio De Hoy. I was dropping him off at JFK airport so he could catch a flight back to Florida after doing a concert for our church the night before. He gave an amazing illustration about the Olympic superstar Michael Phelps. He mentioned the amount of calories Michael Phelps eats each day. I believe it is somewhere in the eight thousand–calorie range. Most people on average consume about fifteen hundred to twenty-five hundred if they stay away from fast food that day. The amazing thing is how lean this swimmer is despite eating so many calories every day. The reason he stays so lean is that his training guards him from the effects of ingesting so many calories. If average people ate that much food, they would see horrible results. They would look and feel out of shape in no time. It would be obvious to everyone that they were caught up in an eating habit that was detrimental to their health. Michael Phelps has gotten his body into such condition that exposure to an unprecedented amount of food had no ability to change the way he looked.

Omar went on to say that we as Christians need to do the same thing. We need to train ourselves so well that when we are exposed to temptations, challenges, and the sins of old, we will not be dragged down. We need to be spiritually fit to the point that exposure to the enemy's attempts to drag us down will do nothing. If we take this training for granted—if we ignore this idea of continuing to grow in Christ—the temptations will catch up to us, and the end result will be as obvious as an average person eating eight thousand calories a day.

If we think we are able to live a righteous life and put no effort into it, we only fool ourselves. It's kind of like the dad who thinks he can still play ball like he did in high school, only to find the years of lying on the couch have changed him from the inside out. His back hurts, his breathing is bad, and when he tries to run, an alarm goes off on the inside like a four-alarm fire has just been sounded. In no time at all, his body tells him, "You can't do what you did when you were a kid." Spiritually and biblically, we cannot rely on doing bare-bones Christianity to carry us through the rough and tough world that is always trying to tear us away from Christ.

Let's look at the second trap that says doing enough things as a child will qualify you to be able to enter heaven despite choices you make in life as you get older. The problem with this way of believing is that some feel serving God is a childish phase and when you get older, you have to deal with real life, like marriage, children, work, and taxes. Who has time to go to church when I've got to put food on the table and get that mortgage paid?

Listen, I live on Long Island where mortgages, rents, and taxes are off the charts. Most couples in our church are forced to both have full-time jobs to make ends meet. Life is kind of, "You work to live." At the end of the day, it would be easy for them to justify not attending God's house or not getting involved in God's kingdom because they are just too busy. The excuse of, "I used to serve God like you when I was a kid" would work out quite conveniently and seem to be "right on" in our own way of thinking. How many times have I heard, "I was an altar boy" or "I used to go to that church"?

It's amazing. It's as if some people think that they have found a new formula to get to heaven. They feel that as a child they did x, y, and z, and now they are covered. They feel that the few years of Bible instruction they received in religion class or Sunday school is enough to get them by for life. It's like saying that after third grade, education is useless—that there is no reason to go to school because there is nothing left for you to learn. It is like saying you have enough education, and it's time to look toward more-important things. How successful are people in our society who don't have more than a third-grade education? Not many; in fact, very few make it at all. What about the Bible? Listen to these words written by John the beloved:

> *This is love for God: to obey his commands.*
> *(1 John 5:3)*

How can you obey commands you don't even know about? What makes us think we can enter God's kingdom if we don't even know what He is asking us to do?

If I took a survey of Long Islanders and asked how many loved Jesus, I believe the response would be pretty good considering today's day and age. If I held their idea of loving Jesus against the Bible's definition of loving Jesus, the number of people who would truly be known by God to love Him would be significantly low.

That breaks my heart, but I can only imagine how it makes the Creator of life feel.

Relying on what you did as a child to qualify you to receive eternal life is about as effective as the guy who curled his sand-filled weights a few times and thought he would have twenty-two-inch, rock-hard, and really vascular arms. It just does not meet the standard of God's requirements.

Imagine if you just got married. You made your vows, went on a honeymoon, and then came home to your new house. The next day, you didn't really talk to your wife anymore. In fact, you never came home and didn't do anything for or with her anymore because you were caught up with other stuff and were just too busy to be bothered. Of course, if you needed your wife, you talked to her because she was the best help you could find, but other than a once-every-other-year cry for assistance, you didn't bother with her. Guess what? You would not have a marriage; you would have a divorce letter in your mail.

Maybe this analogy will help you see how we are treating God when we simply rely on the things we did when we were kids instead of building a healthy, long-lasting relationship that will flourish as it ages. God's standard of living for Him does not get satisfied in one day, year, or decade. Rather, He is asking for our whole life. This is an everyday love affair. God yearns to talk to us, teach us, guide us, etc. There is not, nor will there ever be, anything more important in life then getting to know the Lord and to have no other gods before Him. Remember, this life is a marathon, not a sprint. Jesus is looking for those who finish this race called Christianity even stronger then when they s t a r t e d .

> *Therefore, since we are surrounded by such a great cloud of witnesses, let us throw off everything that hinders and the sin that so easily entangles, and let us run with perseverance the race marked out for us. Let us fix our eyes on Jesus, the author and perfecter of our faith. (Heb. 12:1–2)*

Take a look at yourself. As a person who may claim to be spiritual or even religious, are you relying on things you learned in the past or are you learning from God every day. Remember, simply being spiritual does not mean you are in good standing with the Lord. The apostle Paul pointed this out to a group of philosophers and thinkers when he was in A t h e n s.

> *Men of Athens! I see that in every way* you are very *religious. For as I walked around and looked carefully at your objects of worship, I even found an altar with this inscription: TO AN UNKNOWN GOD. Now what you worship as something unknown I am going to proclaim to you. (Acts 17:22b–23)*

After this, Paul went on to explain who Christ is and how they needed to know Him and Him alone to be saved from their sins. They had plenty of information, rituals, and traditions. They acted pretty good, but being spiritual or religious was not the key to entering the kingdom of God.

In another chapter, we will talk about the only true source of learning, but for now, what are you relying on? Are you acting like a Christian? Do you carry a copy of an insurance policy that can never be cashed in? After reading this, please ask yourself if you used to look like a person who followed Jesus and have been deceived into thinking you are fine when it comes to eternal life. If you say you never did, then I invite you to ask Him to be your Savior, as stated in the beginning of this chapter under the "Godliness" section. If you remember what it was like and you want to get back to where you need to be, then just talk to the God who is waiting for you with open arms. By the way, those are the biggest and strongest guns you'll ever be embraced by!

Things to Ponder:

1) Did you get a clear understanding of the term *born again*? Did you know that it was Jesus who said we need to have this change of heart in John 3:3?

2) How hard are you willing to work to fulfill your dreams? Are you willing to work that hard to honor the Lord?

3) Do you think God will be impressed with bare-bones minimum type of living for Him?

4) Are you training yourself to be spiritually stronger then you were yesterday?

5) Rate yourself from one being the least and one hundred the most, how much of your life does God have control of?

CHAPTER 3

YOU ARE WHAT YOU EAT

—Ludwig Andreas Feuerbach

Give us today our daily bread. (Matt. 6:11)

Physical Training:

Food, glorious food ... Just the mention of it sounds good! I remember that when I was growing up I was told on several occasions by those who knew me best that I should check to see if I had a tapeworm because I ate so much and never seemed to get full.

I don't know if it's true, but many times I've heard it takes twenty minutes for your brain to get the message to your stomach that it is full, or is it the other way around? Either way, my philosophy as an American-Italian is to get as much in my belly during those twenty minutes as possible. That's why this chapter on diet is so important. Diet will make or break your success as a bodybuilder.

Walk into any gym. Take a good look around. What I like to do is try to imagine how some of those monsters who lift the mega-weight would look if they lost a decent percentage of their body fat. Inside every committed weightlifter, there is a physique that will stun people if the weightlifter would only change his diet. It's right there, just a few inches off the surface with one thing in the way: *fat*. It's that coating of stuff that makes us look flat, smooth, and out of shape. Now granted, there is a way to eat for off-season training that is very different from the diet used to prepare for a show, but discipline in eating needs to be constant or that hard work in the gym becomes, very often, just another good workout lost in the wind.

When I got ready for my first show, I was ready to eat whatever I was told. My diet consisted of oats with raisins, egg whites, tuna, fruit, chicken, salad, and bananas. Oh, I can't forget one and a half gallons of water a day. Eat like this for seven to twelve weeks, and you will see a difference. I guarantee it. I actually had learned the oven-stuffer roaster principle during this first preparation for competition. My innie bellybutton became an outtie when my body fat got really low. From then on out, I knew I was ready for a show when my bellybutton popped, much like you can tell that an oven-stuffer roaster chicken is done when it's little plastic popper gets hot enough and pops out.

Changing my diet was probably one of the most difficult things I had ever done. It was a constant struggle to not eat my favorite foods, like chicken parm with angel hair pasta, chocolate cake, cookies, and Taco Bell. Trying not to eat them and to eat food that was bland and boring was not easy. I ate the same food at the same time every day. I had a friend who would just do Sweet and Low shots just to have a taste of sweetness.

I remember for one show I would wake up and eat about three cups of Nabisco Shredded Wheat—and that's dry, with no milk. I'm not talking about Frosted Mini-Wheats—just the stuff that looks like hay. After the fourth week, I thought I could actually taste the sugar in the grains of wheat. It was difficult, to say the least. Cooking egg whites at home and then bringing them to work and nuking them again for lunch was no picnic either.

One thing was for sure—if you had reservations about being a bodybuilder, the diet would sift you out. If I hadn't been so passionate about getting better and if I hadn't truly loved the sport I was in, then there was no way I would have sacrificed so much. I was passionate about competing on stage, and the only way to get there was to have a strict diet! There was the occasional guy who competed who everyone couldn't stand. I remember in my second show a guy from my gym competed in a different weight class but was truly ripped. You could see every vein and muscle fiber bursting through his skin. When I asked him about the diet, he replied, "I eat what I want. I'm naturally ripped." What I wouldn't have done for a metabolism like that.

The morning of competition is such an electric feeling. The atmosphere is awesome. Hundreds of people gather in a school or hotel, and then you register for the contest. You get weighed in and get your stage number, and it is all part of the moment. One thing you could never do before the time to "pump up" came was truly size up your competition. Everyone stayed covered up till the last minute. You didn't want to give the competition a peek at what they were up against.

I have to say that I was stunned at what a difference a pair of sweats and a hooded jacket made on some people. During a bodybuilding show, especially an amateur one where most people don't know each other, you cannot and must not judge a book by its cover. Those you thought would be awesome many times looked bloated or flat. Then, just as often, the guy who looked like nothing covered up was causing everyone to gasp over how ripped he got for the show. It didn't take long for everyone to know who kept the diet and who didn't.

I'll never forget how I felt watching a guy who, during the prejudging, got everyone's attention. Not only did he not tan, shave off his body hair, or know how to pose, but he was also really out of shape. Maybe he worked out, but you would never have known by the way he looked. Some people giggled, and some were insulted that he actually was wasting their time being up there. I just felt bad for him and figured someone probably told him to give it a shot. There was no mistaking it; a disciplined diet was not a part of his lifestyle.

The day of a show has two big payoffs. The first one is that all that you work so hard for is coming to a head. You get to show off all you have worked so hard to achieve. You pose before the judges and then in the evening pose before a large crowd. If you place in the top five, you get a nice trophy. Like I said in chapter 1, as long as I gave my all and did my best, I never left a show unhappy with what happened.

The second payoff is that you are going to come off the diet for at least a few days. On the day of my first show, I made sure to bring with me a Hershey's Bar-None candy bar. I don't think they make that anymore, but being a chocoholic, I needed to have that taste in my mouth. My taste buds were going to do a dance, and my feet would soon follow along. That was the best-tasting food I have ever had in my life. Immediately after the show, my dad and I went to a pizzeria in the city somewhere. I ate three slices of pizza and a calzone. Now, I'm not exaggerating—I felt my stomach start to stretch, and it hurt, but the pleasure of what I was tasting was so immense I couldn't stop.

You have to remember, I was eating the same thing every day for about seven weeks before my first show. My stomach was a food-digesting machine. My stomach was tighter than it had ever been in all of my other attempts to get ripped. My actual stomach, that thing that holds our food, was not used to anything going in there except what was described in the beginning of this chapter. I do believe I could have actually hurt myself if I let it go much further. For the next couple of days, I ate some awesome make-up foods. That's food you have to eat because you missed them so much. I had to hit the fast-food joints so I could eat the stuff I saw the commercials pushing while I was on the strict, get ready for the show diet. You may not believe me on this one, but in just two days' time I gained seventeen pounds. That's right—I jumped from 157 to 174 in two days.

One thing people love to do is try to get you to fall off your diet. I don't know why this happens. Whether it's during your show-time prep diet or a good and healthy off-season diet, people love to temp you to cheat. It's like being around an Italian mother. She won't take no for an answer, and you are forced to eat three plates of lasagna. Many times that situation is simply a cook who loves to get a great reaction over his or her delicious creations. Other times people just try to lure you away, if only for a moment, to taste the forbidden fruit of food that you try so hard to avoid.

I think I've figured out why this happens. So many people have a tough time dealing with their weight. They try to eat healthy and fall off the wagon time and time again. Figure they gain about five pounds of fat a year. Add up ten years and now he or she is fifty pounds overweight. The moment you eat the food that is not on your healthy list is a pleasing moment for these people. For that short period of time, they don't have to feel guilty watching you diet while they keep up a bad habit. If you cheat for the moment, they are not reminded of the issue they really need to address. When you are in really good shape, it makes some people—not all—feel self-conscious about themselves when you're around them. It's odd that the one way they can sort of justify what they are consuming is because you're having it with them. I would basically try to explain myself to the best of my ability, and if I saw it was really irritating them, I would just take a taste to keep the peace.

One of the reasons diet for me was so important was because

I always remained a natural bodybuilder. I did not use drugs to manipulate my body fat or take pills that were illegal to lose my water and look more ripped and vascular. I'm totally honest about this point because I have no reason to lie. Since I did loads of drugs in high school, I'm actually surprised I didn't use performance-enhancing drugs to get an edge.

I remember one friend from Gold's Gym in Lynbrook telling me that I wouldn't have to really worry about diet, that I could eat what I felt like and still be ripped like him, if I took the stuff he was on. As enticing as it was, I never did it. I would have to guess that although I did a lot of stuff that could have harmed me for the sake of a good time, I did it all without my dad around. Training and getting seriously into the bodybuilding scene with my dad was most likely the reason for me staying clean.

I remember one time he had told me that I let him down because I quit the varsity football team in Valley Stream. I really didn't want to hear him say that again, and I knew using steroids would have dropped the level of pride he had in me at the time. Either way, I'm glad I never did it and have plenty of health coming my way as a result. Besides, I look at my dad today, who is in his early sixties and he still has a better build than anyone we know his age.

Since I chose the natural route, I got to work with Joe Jackson, former New York Jet and Minnesota Viking, on anti-drug campaigns in Queens. He allowed me to talk during a school rally about the negative effects of steroids and how staying natural for bodybuilding as well as athletics was the only choice to make. Staying natural meant my diet would have to be watched closely if I was going to have any success and that it would be a harder road as well.

I'm really amazed at the human body and how it responds to what we eat. You can literally change the entire appearance of your physique based on what you choose to put or not put in your mouth. As the old saying goes, "You are what you eat." From a bodybuilding standpoint, truer words were never spoken.

Godliness:

In Matthew 4, an incredible part of Jesus' life is revealed. As soon as He was baptized and His time to start His ministry on earth had come, He was tempted by the Devil. In fact, the Devil attacked Jesus in three different ways. The first of these temptations tells us a tremendous amount about who God longs for us to be.

> *Then Jesus was led by the Spirit into the desert to be tempted by the devil. After fasting forty days and forty nights, he was hungry. The tempter came to him and said, "If you are the Son of God, tell these stones to become bread." Jesus answered, "It is written: 'Man does not live on bread alone, but on every word that comes from the mouth of God.'"* (Matt. 4:1–4)

In this passage that Jesus was quoting from Deuteronomy 8:3, He gave a strong reminder to all who would hear about His ministry for centuries to come. This is the first thing that came His way. He hadn't healed a single person. He hadn't turned water into wine. He hadn't even preached a message yet. The first instruction we hear from the lips of the Savior is that we as men should not only remember that it is important to feed our bodies, but we must also feed our souls.

Did you get that? Just as the body needs food to live, so the spirit needs God's Word to live. Remember that Jesus said man does not live by bread alone. The word *live* is key. He is saying that by taking food into us, we live; we exist. In the same way, He said that we *live* by every word that proceeds from the mouth of God. If we do not have God's Word in us, then we are not living; we do not have life. You cannot separate God from His Word. If you are His child, then you must know Him. The only way to know Him is to have a steady diet of the commands of the living God. Also consider this point. Jesus is stating that we must live according to what He says. In other words, we must obey those commands, not just learn them. As the Bible says in James:

> **Do not merely listen to the word, and so deceive yourselves. Do what it says. (James 1:22)**

This is important because Romans 10 tells us faith comes by hearing the Word. Now that does not mean that once you hear, you automatically have faith. It means that by hearing God's Word, you have the opportunity to believe what is written and thus find yourself being one who now has faith in the Word of God. By hearing the Word, a challenge is brought to the hearers' minds as to whether they want to follow Jesus. This decision can end up in rejection or faith. Jesus is looking for people to live for Him, and that life can only be accomplished by having knowledge of and faith in Christ.

When Christians start to get this understanding of how important a steady diet of the Word of God is, they will be on a road to victory in this life. In fact, Jesus instantly shows us how important and how powerful the Word of God is when it comes to spiritual assaults of the enemy on God's children. How did Jesus handle this time of temptation? Did He call fire down on Satan? Did He call the angels, as He was tempted by the Devil to do? Did He use His authority as God and tell the Devil to flee? No, Jesus used the Word. He used Scripture to combat the temptations and lies of the Devil. What that says to me immediately is Jesus put this enemy of ours in his place by doing what we have the privilege of doing today: standing on the promises of God's Word. It tells me that the Word of God is exactly as the writer of Hebrews says:

> **For the word of God is living and active. Sharper than any double-edged sword, it penetrates even to dividing soul and spirit, joints and marrow; it judges the thoughts and attitudes of the heart. (Heb. 4:12)**

Friends, just as diet can make or break your success as a bodybuilder, so your spiritual diet can make or break your walk with Jesus. In direct contrast to a gym filled with people who have all their potential being robbed from them because of poor diet, so the church is also filled with people who are missing their potential because they keep missing their daily bread. When it comes to food, if you eat garbage long enough, you will look like garbage. If instead of eating, fruits, vegetables, fish, lean meat, whole grains, etc., you eat Twinkies, pizza, fast food, etc., you will look like it. It's only a matter of time before it shows. This is my observation with many people who try to follow Christ yet try to live off only occasionally taking in a good, healthy portion of His Word. The rest of the time they allow themselves to read, watch, or be exposed to things that are garbage, and trust me, it starts to show. It can come from bad spiritual teaching:

> *For the time will come when men will not put up with sound doctrine. Instead, to suit their own desires, they will gather around them a great number of teachers to say what their itching ears want to hear." (2 Tim. 4:3)*

Or it can come from other sources, such as what we read in this verse of the Psalms:

I will set before my eyes no vile thing. (Ps. 101:3)

Here we are told to not even allow things to be put in front of our eyes that would be considered vile in the eyes of the Lord. It's amazing how many individuals who claim to follow Christ just ignore this passage and usually for the sake of entertainment. Movies, magazines, and the Internet are filled with things Jesus was on the cross for. Yet instead of not putting any of these vile things before our eyes, we are dining on them with a ravenous appetite. No wonder so many people are desensitized to violence and vulgarity. It's part of their everyday e n t e r t a i n m e n t.

If only we were taking in a healthy portion of God's Word and letting Him fill our hearts with what pleases Him. I could imagine the difference I would see in the lives of so many if they would just start to change their diets. What happens is most of these people will take in the garbage all week and then get to church and feel guilty and have a kind of spiritual bulimia going on. They get it all out at the altar and receive forgiveness. They feel better for a moment until the urge to take in what is vile consumes them.

Without a steady intake of "every word that proceeds from the mouth of God," a Christian is going to have a very hard time fighting those temptations Jesus dealt with. If we do not have God's Word to guide us, how will we be able to follow Paul's words to the Philippian church?

> *Finally, brothers, whatever is true, whatever is noble, whatever is right, whatever is pure, whatever is lovely, whatever is admirable—if anything is excellent or praiseworthy—think about such things. (Phil. 4:8)*

Paul is telling us that our minds should be filled with God's plans and desires—that we should be contemplating what He would want us to do. We should reflect on the testimonies of others and the answers to prayers we have offered up to Him. This is difficult to do when we choose to put things that are vile to God in our hearts instead of the things God has lovingly done to save us and bless us. If we are going to live a life of victory, it's going to take God's Word in our hearts to make it happen.

> *I have hidden your word in my heart that I might not sin against you. (Ps. 119:11)*

It's only with the words of our God seared into the heart of each person who claims to love Him that we will be able to live full lives for our King. I want to be a law-abiding citizen both in America and in the kingdom of God. It's my business to find out what the law is so I may live by it. Being naive to the law may get you a pass the first time in this country, but it's not the police officer's responsibility to let you get off with a warning just because you didn't know the speed limit. He has every right to give you a ticket if he feels like it.

Friends, simply saying, "I didn't know" will not get you a pass in God's kingdom. We need to be proactive in learning His Word so we can know what is good and what pleases our Lord. Then we can start making choices that will be pleasing to Him and not sin against Him. Please remember that a bodybuilder may have a strong knowledge of what he needs to eat to get the look of a competitor, but if he never eats it, the knowledge does him no good. So it is with the Word of God. You can read it, but if you do not get it in you, as Psalm 119:11 says, it will do you no good. In fact, read Psalm 119 in its entirety. Listen to how many times the writer talks about God's Word and what it means to Him. We should be so in love with the wisdom that comes from the mouth of the Creator.

Now the type of temptation we face is not exactly like the one Jesus went through. Most likely the Devil will use someone else to try to tempt you to stay away from eating the bread of life. Just like when people would try to get me to eat "cheat food," there will be people who will try to get you to cheat on your spiritual diet. You need to be very careful who you choose to surround yourself with. If the people you spend lots of time with have no use for God and His Word, they will very likely try to talk you out of having a steady diet of His Word. They don't understand the importance of getting closer with the Lord. Your godly lifestyle will be in direct contrast to their worldly living. Your presence will remind them of their sin. It will be uncomfortable for them to hear about or even see your lifestyle of godliness. You need to be very careful in this area. You don't want to set yourself apart from all people who don't know the Lord because then you have no chance to help them find God. You just need to know when their influence on you is more effective than your influence on them. Listen to what God's Word says about this:

> Do not be misled: "Bad company corrupts good character." (1 Cor. 15:33)

People who eat forbidden fruit (things that are sinful in the eyes of the Lord) very often have a knowledge of God to some degree. They choose to satisfy their own flesh and feed on what they desire instead of what God yearns to give them. It's amazing how the same principle applies to fruit and candy. Candy comes in an attractive wrapper and tastes good at first, but too much will get you sick and/ or cause you to gain weight, and often you regret having it. Fruit, however, is tasty and healthy, and if you eat too much you never really have a negative result unless you have sugar problems. That's the comparison Paul makes between the fruit of the Spirit and the lust of the flesh. The contrast is found in Galatians 5:19–23:

> *The acts of the sinful nature are obvious: sexual immorality, impurity and debauchery; idolatry and witchcraft; hatred, discord, jealousy, fits of rage, selfish ambition, dissensions, factions and envy; drunkenness, orgies, and the like. I warn you, as I did before, that those who live like this will not inherit the kingdom of God. But the fruit of the Spirit is love, joy, peace, patience, kindness, goodness, faithfulness, gentleness and self-control. Against such things there is no law.*

Not only do they choose to do things their way, but they are strong supporters of those who would join them in their sinfully gluttonous road to destruction.

> *Furthermore, since they did not think it worthwhile to retain the knowledge of God, he gave them over to a depraved mind, to do what ought not to be done. They have become filled with every kind of wickedness, evil, greed and depravity. They are full of envy, murder, strife, deceit and malice. They are gossips, slanderers, God-haters, insolent, arrogant and boastful; they invent ways of doing evil; they disobey their parents; they are senseless,*

faithless, heartless, ruthless. Although they know God's righteous decree that those who do such things deserve death, they not only continue to do these very things but also approve of those who practice them. *(Rom. 1:28–32)*

I need to emphasize the importance God puts on His creation, knowing what He has given us in the Bible. In fact, it was a Bible school teacher of mine who reminded me of this true point. God uses five words to describe the creation of the stars:

He also made the stars. (Gen. 1:16)

If Hollywood made the movie of creation, they would have been so elaborate in their presentation of the "creating of the stars"—the explosions, the great light, the tossing into their place from the hand of God. Simply written, God only used five words to talk about it, yet He wrote the entire Bible to tell you how much He loves you! That's how much you mean to Him and how important His Word is for us to know. Listen to Luke's opinion of a special group of people who loved to learn God's Word:

Now the Bereans were of more noble character than the Thessalonians, for they received the message with great eagerness and examined the Scriptures every day to see if what Paul said was true. (Acts 17:11)

How about the longevity and importance of Jesus' description of the Scriptures?

Heaven and earth will pass away, but my words will never pass away. (Luke 21:33)

In fact, the Bible makes it clear to us that this Word is more than just good penmanship or historical literature:

> *In the beginning was the Word, and the Word was*
> *with God, and the Word was God. (John 1:1)*

> *I am the living bread that came down from heaven.*
> *If anyone eats of this bread, he will live forever.*
> *(John 6:51)*

John is making us totally see that Jesus is the Word! Jesus is the bread of life! When we study these precious Scriptures, when we read the ancient texts penned by some forty different authors over some fifteen hundred years, this is not simply history. This is His story! If you say that you do not regularly live by every word that proceeds from the mouth of God, you are saying you don't have time to get to know the Jesus who died for you and provides the only way to eternal life.

I get sad about this point just like when I got sad about that guy who was on stage and you knew he just didn't belong. You could tell he didn't diet, and although he may have tried a little good eating here and there, nobody was fooled, and he stuck out like a sore thumb.

People who first learn about Jesus and start their relationship have a reason to say they have yet to do the things that please the Lord. They have yet to stop looking at the vile or think about the holy things of God. They just don't know yet. They learn as they go, and then they are expected to change as God teaches them. That's what happens to disciples. They learn the way they should go.

If after two or three years, there is no change, it's because one of two things: either they haven't learned the Word of God or they haven't let the Word of God get into their heart. Regardless of the reason, this person sticks out in God's kingdom. Some people get upset with them; others may show their disappointment by giggling and trying not to offend them. Personally, I just get sad because so much potential is there, yet because they continue to take in the junk, it just stays hidden. As the old saying goes, "You are what you eat." From a biblical standpoint, truer words were never spoken.

Things to Ponder:

1) Have you ever given up anything you enjoy or desire to attain a goal? Could you deny yourself if what you like to do puts a tear in God's eye instead of a smile on His face?

2) Can you truly say you know what the Bible says? Can you truly say you follow the Word of God?

3) Is there anything you may be exposing yourself to that may be making you spiritually sick?

4) What truly rules your heart: God's Word or your desires?

CHAPTER 4
THE TRAINING PARTNER

As iron sharpens iron, so one man sharpens another.
(Prov. 27:17)

Physical Training:

Ever hear this in a gym: "Hey pal, could I get a spot? Can I get some help? Can you give me a hand?" This is the request of someone who knows he or she is about to attempt something that is most likely beyond his or her ability to control. It may be a guy going for a max rep on the bench. Maybe it is someone who is doing a really heavy set of squats. Maybe it's an endurance set, and even though the weight is light, before the set is done, the person wants to do some negatives and really exhaust and thoroughly attack the muscle he or she is training. A negative is when you can no longer push the weight so your partner picks it up for you and you simply resist it from coming down on you. Basically you fight gravity because that's all the strength you have left.

Whatever the need is, a spotter can make the difference between a good workout and a great one! It's humbling to ask someone you don't know to help you out, but putting your pride aside to be sure you're safe is a must. Some may settle on doing it alone because they are afraid to ask or because someone may think he or she is weak, maybe even annoying. So be it. The need for the spot and the benefits it brings is more important than getting hurt or thought of in a negative way. Besides, if someone is bothered by you asking for a spot, no problem. There is always someone else.

From the idea of getting help from someone in the gym to assist you with moving those mountains of steel, I've learned a couple of truths. The first thing is that not everyone is able to give you a spot. There are those who you can use to help you blast out a few extra reps on the curling bar, but if someone was going to spot me squatting, it was a different story. Anyone can help you when your health is not on the line.

I remember a time when two friends of mine decided that we should all work out together. Normally I wouldn't do this because it would take too long between sets, but I thought I'd give it a shot. We were doing triceps, and the exercise was lying down nose breakers. One guy did the movement, one guy spotted, and the other watched and rested. It was my turn to rest, and my buddy doing his set was getting fatigued. As he was slowing down, I noticed our other friend looking in the mirror and staring at his triceps as they were now pumped from the few sets we had done. He was posing away and flexing hard, but he forgot he was supposed to be spotting our other buddy. Well, my friend who was doing the exercise gave out, and the bar came crashing down on his forehead. Our friend who was checking himself out in the mirror heard the sudden cry of pain and raced to help lift the bar. He was apologizing as he was getting yelled at by our friend with the new red line across his forehead. I was just laughing and thought, *I'll never train with three guys again.* I also saw the difference between a casual spot and a real partner.

I've never seen anyone get crushed while doing standing curls. Squats are a different story. You need to know how to hold the person squatting; wrapping your arms around him is much safer and easier than trying to lift the bar on his shoulders! You never ask someone who looks lost in the gym to help when you can truly get hurt if the spotter is unskilled at assisting others on big lifts. How much help to give during a spot is also important. Many times people gave me some help and basically ruined a great set because they did the work and never let me really do the rep.

Not only is having the right guy spot you important, but I've also found out that there is a significant difference between a spotter and a training partner. The spotter is just some person who is around at the time. A training partner is someone who knows not only how to give you the right spot but also how to push you to places you could never get to on your own. This is a person you trust who can motivate you and really help you get to the goals you have much more quickly than on your own. In my life, I've only had a handful of people who I've called my training partner. The reason is this: your partners can make or break your success in the gym. If they slack or waste time, it will affect you. But if they are hard core, intense, and challenging, you will have one of the best workouts of your life.

My first partner was my dad. Later in life, it became my best friend Pete. As I was in competition mode, a friend named Allen who was also a US Marine helped get me ready for my third show. Now, I've had others train me, but these were the only guys I truly trained regularly with. Not only did they push me, but I pushed them. The most gut-wrenching, exhausting, and intense workouts I've ever had were with these guys. I consider them war buddies. We have some good memories of training together.

When you partner with someone in that way, you form a bond that is not easily forgotten. When you push each other so much that you can barely walk out of a gym or turn the steering wheel of your car, you form a connection that is not quickly forgotten. You keep each other focused and remind each other of the goal in front of you. A training partner is not someone you choose on a whim. You need to be sure that this person will be committed, faithful, and dedicated to the vow you have made to one another about getting to the gym at all costs. You must know that he or she will be there for you and you can count on him or her. If you're not motivated and don't feel like lifting, your partner will get your head into it. If you feel like you're exhausted from work, he'll tell you that someone else is there working harder then you to get first place at the next show. A dedicated, loyal training partner is worth his or her weight in gold.

When choosing a training partner, I have a few beliefs that are totally matters of opinion. The first is this: I don't need my training partner yelling at me or insulting me to try to get me motivated. You know the type. They say things like, "Come on, lift that bar. My grandmother can do better than that." I don't know where the idea of insulting people to get them to try harder came from. It's like the sadistic football coach who would call his players ladies and make fun of them if they didn't execute the tackle or follow their assignment. Telling me I'm a waste or that my effort is embarrassing does not make me want to push harder; it would make me want to get a new partner. Thankfully the guys I lifted with regularly understood the power of speaking life, not death. Sure, there were times of yelling and saying, "Don't give up. Don't you quit on me," but that's understandable and acceptable. I will always respond better to comments like, "You can do it. Come on, give it all you got! Let's go!" Saying things to build me up did just that. It built me up. Saying things to tear me down would tear me down. Actually, it would just turn me off!

The other important part about choosing training partners is that they should not be far away from you in strength, dedication, etc. In other words, you shouldn't have to hold them by the hand to get through the workout. They most definitely should be able to hold their own. My dad was, until recently, much stronger than I. He gave me the desire to lift and was way ahead of me when we trained together. If anything, I slowed him down. My pal Pete, although he wasn't a bodybuilder, was an animal—six foot three and 250 to 275 pounds. He lifted heavy and motivated really well. My Marine friend Allen was not as strong as me, but what he lacked in strength, he made up for in heart. He was a recruiter for the US Marine Corps and knew how to get me into that "I know I can" mode. Honestly, it was with him that I pushed myself to places I thought I could never get in the gym.

I have been training with free weights for twenty-seven years now. I have had partners, and I've trained on my own. For the last fifteen years or so, it's been a solo act for me. I work out at my house and do what I love to do, and I thank God that I have the discipline to keep it up since I am now in my forties. For many people not having a partner means they work out at random. They do not have the discipline to train on a regular basis because they have no accountability to get it done. They may work out for a few months, but then the weights get dusty because life gets busy. That gym membership is not being used, and nobody even realizes you haven't been around. It's a sad thing to love something so much and yet let it get covered in dust and cobwebs with no one to blame but yourself. A personal trainer is a great idea for those who can afford it, but I believe that *for most people,* a great training partner is the difference between going through the motions and actually reaching your goals.

Godliness:

Ever hear this in a church: "Do you think we can talk? I need your help! Can I meet with you for a little while? I need to tell you something." This is the cry of someone who is facing something in life he or she understands is too much to handle. The response to recognizing this point in one's life leads us to reach out to someone for assistance with things we cannot take care of ourselves. Just like the gym, where you can find a spotter or a training partner, the Bible has given us advice on life and how to find the help we need to maximize our spiritual growth.

Comparable to the spotter in the gym, God has blessed us with compassionate people whose wisdom to counsel or encourage us during that time is much needed. These people are able to help in various ways:

> *Now you are the body of Christ, and each one of you is a part of it. And in the church God has appointed first of all apostles, second prophets, third teachers, then workers of miracles, also those having gifts of healing, those able to help others, those with gifts of administration, and those speaking in different kinds of tongues. (1 Cor. 12:27–28)*

> *So in Christ we who are many form one body, and each member belongs to all the others. We have different gifts, according to the grace given us. If a man's gift is prophesying, let him use it in proportion to his faith. If it is serving, let him serve; if it is teaching, let him teach; if it is encouraging, let him encourage; if it is contributing to the needs of others, let him give generously; if it is leadership, let him govern diligently; if it is showing mercy, let him do it cheerfully. (Rom. 12:5–8)*

Notice how God has given to the body so many different types of people to be there for those in the church who may need them. Let's face it: life is harder than the gym, but the principles remain the same. Remember that in the gym, I had to ask for help. Very rarely did people come over to me and ask if I needed the spot. It was nice of them, but if I didn't know them, I would usually say no because I didn't know if they knew what they were doing. We need to be willing to ask for help in life. Jesus has built His church to be there for one another and help each other out in various ways. In order to get this help, we need to be humble enough to be able to ask for the assistance we need. Don't let pride be a factor in keeping you from getting the help Christ wants to give you. Remember these words:

> *For your Father knows what you need before you ask him. (Matt. 6:8)*

> *Until now you have not asked for anything in my name. Ask and you will receive, and your joy will be complete. (John 16:24)*

Just like a spotter, in the church there are those who can handle the small things with you and those who you can trust to handle the heavy loads as well. There will be times when the need you have can be taken care of by someone you know strictly on a Sunday-only relationship. In other words, you have seen them in church and haven't really gotten together but always say hello and are happy to see them when you are in God's house. Please know that there will always be relationships like this in church. It's impossible to be a part of a growing church and having everyone who attends breaking bread around your table. These people may help you with a ride somewhere, giving you a hand carrying something, or even holding your seat when service is full.

There will also be times when you have a heavy load and need to go to someone who you know can handle the news you share with respect, confidence, and integrity. This could be a marital problem, some type of sin, finances, etc. In the gym, I could tell by the shape of the person if he or she could handle the spot I needed. In church, it's the spiritual maturity and Christian lifestyle of a person that determines who could be approached like this. We should always be looking to build one another up as we read:

> *And let us consider how we may spur one another on toward love and good deeds. Let us not give up meeting together, as some are in the habit of doing, but let us encourage one another—and all the more as you see the Day approaching. (Heb. 10:24–25)*

With all that said, there is very big difference between a person who helps you on the spot and an accountability partner who helps you through life. In church we may be called upon to help out people in a many different ways, but not everyone is going to ask you to be accountable to him or her, and neither should you be open to the idea without proper prayer and consideration put into it.

Just like a training partner, an accountability partner is going to help you get to places in your walk with the Lord that you most likely would never have been able to arrive at alone. This is a person who can motivate you and speak not just to you but right into your life. These people look you in the eye and challenge you to step it up and live a holy life that is pleasing and glorifying to the Lord. When you have messed up, you feel horrible telling these people about it—not because they get mad but because you feel like you let them down. They are also people who you can share the highest of moments with, and usually they are the first ones you call to tell good news. They would fit this description very well:

> *As iron sharpens iron, so one man sharpens another. (Prov. 27:17)*

Accountability partners should never tear you down when you make a mistake. They should never be demeaning and insulting. If they are demeaning, then they don't get the meaning! You have to be very open and vulnerable to an accountability partner. Your life is an open book, and for them to take advantage or hurt you when you share your faults, shortcomings, or sins would be devastating. No accountability partner worth having would ever do that. Rather, they would advise you with God's Word, not their opinion. They would build you up and pray for you when you are weak. These people will treasure the fact that you have given them the privilege to know the intimate details of your life and treat the responsibility with trust and respect.

Remember that this person should also be a mature believer who is able to pick you up and not be caused to stumble if you should fall. How could a partner lift you back up if he or she doesn't know how stand alone? Listen to the description of a church leader and the importance Paul puts on maturity as a requirement to lead in the church:

> *Here is a trustworthy saying: If anyone sets his heart on being an overseer, he desires a noble task ... He must not be a recent convert, or he may become conceited and fall under the same judgment as the devil.* (*1 Tim. 3:1, 6*)

It's amazing how often we are encouraged to see the benefits of having someone walk this journey of serving Jesus with us:

> *Though one may be overpowered, two can defend themselves. A cord of three strands is not quickly broken. (Eccles. 4:12)*

When Jesus had fully poured out His life to His twelve disciples, He told them something that must have really melted them inside. Listen to this:

> *I no longer call you servants, because a servant does not know his master's business. Instead,*

> *I have called you friends, for everything that I*
> *learned from my Father I have made known to you.*
> *(John 15:15)*

Imagine the moment. Jesus just told these men that they have gotten to the place where hundreds of other disciples would never get. The twelve were very dear to Him and had a special place in His heart. He also had a special relationship with three disciples that was different from the relationship with the twelve. Peter, James, and John were the ones He took to the mountain where He was transfigured before their eyes. He also brought them to the garden of Gethsemane, where He would eventually be arrested and the suffering would begin. Not only did Jesus love the three, but He also loved the one. Listen to his passage during the Passover meal.

> *After he had said this, Jesus was troubled in spirit*
> *and testified, "I tell you the truth, one of you is*
> *going to betray me." His disciples stared at one*
> *another, at a loss to know which of them he meant.*
> *One of them, the disciple whom Jesus loved, was*
> *reclining next to him. Simon Peter motioned to this*
> *disciple and said, "Ask him which one he means."*
> *Leaning back against Jesus, he asked him, "Lord,*
> *who is it?" (John 13:21–25)*

Look at how Peter, who Jesus was very close to, asked the one who Jesus loved to get the inside scoop for the rest of them. It seems that Jesus had a relationship with John that was even a little deeper and intimate than the three.

Friends, having someone in our lives to help us walk the straight and narrow is critical. Yet there are some figures in the Bible who did not practice this behavior, people like Joseph and Daniel. These guys had no church to attend to be encouraged and no Bible study to learn the Word of God better. They had no pastor to call them to see how they were doing. There was something else they didn't have: a choice. Joseph was sold into slavery and for thirteen years worked faithfully for his owners until he became head of all Egypt under Pharaoh. Daniel was a Jewish captive take into exile and stripped away from his family. We can choose to live for God without getting an accountability partner and merely say we are accountable to the Lord. This is a truth that cannot be overlooked. We will all give an account to God:

> *So then, each of us will give an account of himself*
> *to God. (Rom. 14:12)*

Please keep this simple truth in mind when I emphasize to you the need for an accountability partner. If you say you are accountable to God, you are correct. You will stand before Him, and He will judge you one day for how you lived your life. Simply living with that accountability has caused many people to miss the mark Christ has called us to reach for.

Here is an example. Every time I have seen something on TV that was not appropriate or contained scenes I shouldn't have watched, Jesus was with me. I guarantee that if my accountability partner was in the room with me, the channel would have changed faster than you could say, "Yo, buddy, could I get a spot!" Even knowing they may ask me if I've watched anything ungodly would cause me to change the channel because I don't want to give an account of sin. I would much rather give a report of victory!

Things to Ponder:

1) Do you get easily distracted from what you are supposed to be doing, especially when it comes to helping others?

2) Do you have someone in your life who will be there for you and you know you can count on? Does this person help you walk with God or walk away from God?

3) What may stop you from asking somebody for help?

4) Are you able to be a godly influence in anyone's life?

CHAPTER 5

A FIRM FOUNDATION

Rome was not built in a day.
—Old French Proverb

Unless the LORD builds the house, its builders labor in vain. (Ps. 127:1)

<u>Physical Training</u>

I am now forty-three years of age. My contest days are more than twenty years in the past. Although this book primarily uses the sport of bodybuilding to make its point, I need to take a turn. For the last four years, I have dedicated myself to a new sport that has always had my interest. I decided to start taking boxing lessons. I figured it would be a great way to lose some body fat and start to get in better shape. I had seen guys in the gym hitting the heavy bag, and I figured, "That's got to be more exciting than the treadmill or an elliptical machine." Basically I wanted to do it for cardio purposes. It was actually a tossup between MMA or boxing. I was watching the UFC and realized that both MMA fighters and boxers had a really tight look to their physiques.

It was September of '07. My daughter Gianna had just started going to kindergarten and had to start taking the bus to school. My wife took her to the bus stop most of the time, but on occasion, I was more than happy to see her off. On one of those mornings, I met a man whose son was also taking the bus for the first time. The man's name was Rob Martinez, and we got to talking. I could tell he was a dedicated weightlifter, and in the midst of one of our conversations, we started to discuss the fight game. It turned out that Rob was not only the manager of a large gym in our town, but he is also a professional boxer. Well, that made up my mind for me. My wife bought me four sessions of boxing with Rob for Christmas that year, and I've been hooked ever since.

Like anything else you do for the first time, you can only guess how much effort it's going to take to do well. To be honest, I had no idea what I was in for. Let me take a second to describe Rob to you. He's about five foot ten and weighs 240 pounds. He's all muscle and works out with about 405 on the bench. He comes from the Bronx, which in my book makes him naturally tough. Despite his size, he is deceivingly fast with his hands, and he can probably hit a guy three or four times before he thinks of covering up.

To be honest, Rob was exactly what I needed. This is the big difference between a training partner and a person who can build you a firm foundation. Although the training partner can be both, it was just not the case for me. The trainer was a guy who mentored me. He was a guy who had tasted the fruit of doing what I could only dream about. A trainer is a person who helps you build a foundation like the one he has stood on himself for a long time. Since Rob was a pro boxer, he knew what it took not just to have a great workout but to be able to reach the heights of inner conditioning that would lead to a solid foundation.

Growing up, I was always the guy who stuck out from the rest of my group when it came to physical fitness. I was honored when people would ask me for advice on diet or if I could make them a workout plan to help them out. It meant they looked to me to be an inspiration and that I was good at what I did. Although it is an honor to be asked these favors, there is one problem: who's going to get me to improve? In other words, if I was the guy who was giving everyone advice, pushing them in the gym, and pouring out motivation, who was going to do this for me? Most of my life has been spent doing things on my own and having to self-motivate. Then came Rob.

I thought I was going to learn how to punch, hit a speed bag, and jump rope—you know, all the stuff you saw Muhammad Ali do. Well, let's get something straight. Before you learn how to fight, you need to be *able* to learn how to fight. My coach quickly showed me that unless you have a solid foundation, you will never be able to stand toe to toe with anyone. In boxing, you quickly realize that if your stamina, endurance, and conditioning are lacking, then you're an easy target for your opponent. No matter how tough you are or how long your reach, if you have poor conditioning, you will most likely lose. In fact, you may have great boxing skills, but if you cannot hold your hands up or if you have no gas left in the tank to throw your punches, you'll be the guy kissing the canvas in no time at all.

I quickly learned that although I used the elliptical for half an hour three times a week and trained with weights three to four times a week, I may have looked okay, but I had no foundation when it came to going the distance. As Rob would say, "Game on." I started doing squat thrusts, running up flights of steps, bunny hops (very evil), lunges, medicine ball training, crazy pushups at weird angles, ab work that would cause me to spit all over, etc. Then there is the punching of the focus pads or punch mitts. If you have no stamina, this exercise will last about twenty seconds. How about hitting the heavy bag with continuous one and two punches so the bag is lifting up in the air and you can't let it come down until the coach says relax? Picture holding five- to eight-pound dumbbells and doing a one-six punching sequence for three minutes without stopping. That burns!

Don't forget the sparring, when you actually get hit back, or the three-minute rounds on the heavy bag, which include slips and combinations. Add in a good dose of running several miles and wind sprints and you have a formula for a boxing foundation. As my coach likes to do, he gets me really fatigued, and then we put the gloves on. It's at that exhausted place where he gets to see what I've truly learned about punching, defending myself, and the instincts I've developed. He also gets to see what kind of heart his fighters have and if they are willing to do whatever it takes to get them to go way past what they could have ever thought they could do.

I have told him we have a love-hate relationship. I hate him for what he's going to make me do, yet I love him for the resultsI'm seeing. I have never been in such great shape. And I've never enjoyed hearing the words, "Game over" as much. This is what Coach says when a boxing session comes to an end. The good thing about "game over" is that you really get a good look at the foundation that has been built up to that point.

Another amazing point about having Rob as a boxing instructor is how even when he is not around, he pushes me. What do I mean? Picture this. I'm in the gym, and Rob, similar to a training partner (which we have discussed) wants me to do a particular movement for two minutes straight. I'm dead by one minute, but I know with him there and his words of encouragement, somehow I'll get to two minutes, even if it's crawling or in slow motion. I'll give him all I got.

Now take a training session at my home. Without Coach around, I may be doing sprints, squat thrusts, hitting the bag, whatever. In my head, when I start to get weak, I hear his voice. At moments when I can just stop and no one would see, he's talking to me. It's amazing how far a person will go when this voice is in his head. Not only is it his voice that I hear, but I also want him to be proud of my results. I want him to know, by the way I look and the things I improve in, that I've been working hard at it even when he's not around. I want him to know I've been pushing myself and not playing a game with all this time invested but rather taking it very serious.

It was under his guidance that I actually got into the ring for the first time and fought in the master's division. To be honest, I had no idea how I would do, but there was one truth that made me believe in my possible success: the fact that Rob believed in me. You see, his opinion of my abilities catapulted me into believing, "I can do this thing." I know he has the experience, I know he has seen what's out there, and I know he would not want me to get hurt. There is no way he would let me get into the ring if he felt I was not ready. So although I may not know what the competition is like, my coach does, and since he has developed this foundation I now have, trusting his evaluating of the situation is a must for me. It's also an amazing confidence booster to have someone so good at what he does share his confidence in me. Now, unfortunately for me, I was stopped in the second round and lost my first fight. Yet, even with that my coach saw it as an amazing learning tool to help us get back into the ring with that much more knowledge of what to do and *what not to do!*

At this point in my life, my lungs are healthier, my legs are stronger, and my body looks like it did when I was competing in the early '90s. I have started to pick up some boxing skills, and along the way have discovered that without a solid foundation, it is impossible to be successful in boxing. I don't believe there is a more enjoyable moment then when you start to see this foundation coming together. I have graduated from doing squat thrusts for one minute to three minutes. I can fight the heavy bag for twelve three-minute rounds, my jump rope skills have much improved, and I actually landed a couple of punches on Rob the last time

Antony L. Pelella

we sparred. I went from 210 pounds to 175 pounds in about nine months, and to be honest, many people still say, "But you weren't heavy." No, I was not heavy, but I was far from being in shape and having muscle tone. I had no internal foundation to speak of.

You see, when the foundation is there, then the real construction can begin. *The great results of conditioning for stamina and endurance is that you are training the inside. If done right, you have no choice but to see it affect the outside as well.* Like all structures, if the foundation is weak, it's eventually going to collapse. It will topple sooner or later. After nine months of boxing lessons, I was finally able to learn how to box. My time can be used more effectively, and my reward of achieving my goal can start to become a reality. If Rob didn't push me to build my foundation, I would just be another guy hitting a bag. Instead, I'm now a conditioned athlete able to enter into uncharted waters—waters I could have never swam in unless I had a foundation to support me. As I heard one fighter say about the training you need to do to get ready for a fight, "The squeeze is worth the juice."

I couldn't agree more.

Godliness:

It was the early '80s. My parents had been divorced for a while. My dad had gotten remarried, and I now had a baby brother. The family picked up and went to Valley Stream to get a fresh start. I was actually excited to see it happen. I was sad to leave my friends but happy to see what our new home would hold for us as a family. Little did I know it was in this town that my life would totally be changed.

I mentioned to you about my pastor meeting with me and how he had a heart-to-heart talk with me about what I was going to do with my life and my devotion to Jesus. I found out that although I had some knowledge about the Lord, my foundation had cracks all over that prohibited me from building anything that looked like an authentic relationship with Jesus. Those cracks were the sins that I somehow convinced myself were all right and that God would still be okay with me despite my practice of them. This is a pretty scary place to be in life if you ask me. Let me remind you what the Bible says, as I did in chapter 2:

> *But mark this: There will be terrible times in the last days. People will be lovers of themselves, lovers of money, boastful, proud, abusive, disobedient to their parents, ungrateful, unholy, without love, unforgiving, slanderous, without self-control, brutal, not lovers of the good, treacherous, rash, conceited, lovers of pleasure rather than lovers of God—having a form of godliness but denying its power.*
> *(1 Tim. 3:1–5a)*

In fact, God despises this place so much that he says this about those who think they are okay with Him:

> *So, because you are lukewarm—neither hot nor cold—I am about to spit you out of my mouth.*
> *(Rev. 3:16)*

You see, I had heard messages from the pulpits of many churches for years. I had people tell me right from wrong as often as I could remember, but it wasn't until I had the truth put into my face by someone who truly touched my heart that I finally saw the problem. Rev. Steve Milazzo is that man. In the same way Rob Martinez has trained me to build a foundation I can work off of to become a boxer, Pastor Steve taught me how to build a foundation God can finally work off of to be a Christian. Let me describe Pastor Steve to you. He kind of looks like John Travolta. He's very funny and dresses very classy. Pastor Steve does not have a physical appearance that is nearly as intimidating as Rob yet when he walks into a room you know that this is a man with God Given authority! This is a man who I can honestly say I have no problem doing as the early church did with the apostle Paul:

> *Follow my example, as I follow the example of Christ. (1 Cor. 11:1)*

You see, my pastor is what I believe God wants us to see in an example of one who follows Christ with all of his heart, mind soul, and strength. His muscle is demonstrated in his countless hours of prayer and compassion for the lost and dying. His love for the church is never questioned, and his devotion to his wife and children is never in doubt. I say these things not to build him up or even to puff him up but rather to say this is what I needed in my life to be built up the right way. If I was going to have a solid foundation that was truly built on Christ, I was going to need a man like this to show me how to build it.

As mentioned before, it was Pastor Steve who led me to truly understand my need to get my life right with God by confessing my sins and truly believing in my heart that Jesus had risen from the grave.

> *That if you confess with your mouth, "Jesus is Lord," and believe in your heart that God raised him from the dead, you will be saved. (Rom. 10:9)*

At a very impressionable time in my life, God knew I needed someone who could mold me for what God was going to do with me in the years to come. I could have never become a Bible school student, a husband, a father, a pastor, or a true child of God if I had not had his help in building a solid foundation of godly living and biblical principles that stick in my heart to this day. When my eyes were first opened to seeing Jesus for who He really was, I was like a sponge. It was at that point that my pastor took me under his wing and really started to teach me what it meant to be a Christian. *This is very different from my accountability partner in that I was being molded from the ground up as opposed to committing to what I had already believed.*

Whenever I was around Pastor Steve, I was challenged to get my life in order. The amazing thing was that this happened not just by his verbal instructions but simply by observing. I observed how he treated his wife and always spoke positively about her. I saw how he treasured his daughters and loved them more than himself. More than anything, the foundation that he was to teach me about was to have regular communication with the Lord. This is called communion or intimacy with God.

I watched Pastor Steve pray and pray and pray and pray. His heart for prayer would become the staple of my ability to hear the voice of the Lord and finally find out His direction for me in ministry. It's amazing the difference I saw in myself as he built up this foundation in me. He at times spent hours teaching me the Bible all alone. He would have me ask questions and show me how to treat people when we visited them together if they were sick. In a short period of time, I saw myself doing things that when I first came under his wing I never thought I could do. I went from being afraid to pray out loud to leading a young adult group. I went from not knowing where anything was found in the Bible to preparing messages and teaching Sunday school classes. After spending time with him, I realized that what I had in the past was simply a poor excuse of Christianity, and I was so glad that I finally learned how to not just read the Bible but live it.

The amazing thing is that today, when I'm faced with a pressure from this world to sin or get caught up in something that would drag me away from God, I hear his voice. Maybe it's from a message he spoke or a personal time when we were talking about living for the Lord, but I hear his voice.

No, I'm not crazy. It's the same thing that happens when I'm training and hear Rob's voice. It's a voice that pushes me to do the right thing even when no one is around. It's like the message Pastor Steve spoke on having pure eyes in a lust-filled world during a GOD4ME rally here on Long Island. He was talking about the temptations we as men may face, and before a crowd of about eight hundred men, he drew an illustration that to this day keeps me going strong. He said he asks God to give him a picture in his mind of his wife and daughters crying and broken over him possibly doing something like being unfaithful in his marriage. He sees this vision, and it reminds him that there is no momentary pleasure worth causing that kind of pain to his family. I do the same thing to this day. Those words literally scream into my heart each time I can feel my guard dropping and know that temptation is rearing its ugly head.

Remember, just like Rob, Pastor Steve helped me to build the foundation I have. The foundation in this case was not built on exercise but rather is based on the Holy Bible. It is not just having knowledge of the Word but putting that knowledge to work every day of my life.

> *Therefore everyone who hears these words of mine and puts them into practice is like a wise man who built his house on the rock. The rain came down, the streams rose, and the winds blew and beat against that house; yet it did not fall, because it had its foundation on the rock. But everyone who hears these words of mine and does not put them into practice is like a foolish man who built his house on sand. The rain came down, the streams rose, and the winds blew and beat against that house, and it fell with a great crash. (Matt. 7:24–27)*

Rev. Steve Milazzo has helped build in me an ability to see the potential God had for me well before I was able to discover it myself. About sixteen years ago, I was asked to leave my home church and take over the church I currently pastor. It was a shell of what it is today. As my wife and I always have said, "No pay, no people, no parsonage, but lots of potential." That quote was not spoken immediately.

My pastor came with me one dark night, and we stood in that small church together. We prayed together, and he looked at me and said, "Anthony, you can preach here." It was a moment where I knew he was giving me his vote of confidence that I could do what was being asked of me, not just by my superiors but by my Lord. You see, Pastor Steve has done some awesome things as a leader of Bethlehem Assembly of God in Valley Stream. The church has grown by leaps and bounds and continues to be a driving force for the kingdom of God on Long Island. He is a pro in my eyes. To have his vote of confidence made me believe in my call to ministry all the more. To take this church, my wife and I would have to swim in uncharted waters and leave a church, at the time, of about eight hundred people we loved.

At our home church, if there was a problem, we could always turn to those who we were working arm in arm with. Pastor Steve was always a few steps away if you needed him, and to be honest, all less-than-profitable decisions and problems went back to him, so it made our jobs in ministry simple. Now in Medford Assembly of God, a church of three people when we began, we had all the responsibility on our shoulders. I would have to answer for all the decisions we made and handle all problems that would come down the pike. Pastor Steve's words of assurance reminded me of the foundation the Holy Spirit built in me. God used Pastor Steve to equip me for a time such as this, and instead of being just a leader in church, I was going to be a pastor.

After four years of doing ministry under Pastor Steve, I was finally able to start doing ministry on my own. My time can be used more effectively, and my reward of achieving my goal has started to become a reality. If Pastor Steve hadn't pushed me to build a biblical foundation, I would just be another guy going to church. Instead I was a credentialed minister able to sail the uncharted waters of reviving a dying church. In fact, these waters and his mentoring have led us to now be the mother church of two other churches here on Long Island that were going to close. These are waters I could have never swum in unless I had a foundation to support me. As it read on Evander Holyfield's robe before his fight with Mike Tyson, "I can do all things through *Christ* who gives me strength" (Phil. 4:13).

Things to Ponder

1) What kind of spiritual condition are you in? How do you know, and who is really testing you?

2) Is there anyone you can get around who can greatly elevate your walk with God?

3) Have you ever heard the voice of someone you trust speaking to your heart in times of difficulty even when he or she is not around?

4) Are you sure you have a strong foundation? If storms hit you, are you strong and peaceful, or do you come crashing down?

CHAPTER 6

SACRIFICE

Fanatic is a word the lazy use to describe the dedicated.
—Bill Phillips

Therefore, I urge you, brothers, in view of God's mercy, to offer your bodies as living sacrifices, holy and pleasing to God—this is your spiritual act of worship. (Rom. 12:1)

Anthony L. Pelella

Physical Training:

Sometimes being a person who is so committed to accomplishing a goal that is foreign to many can get lonely. The percentage of people who share the same degree of faithfulness to physical fitness that myself or other bodybuilders possess is very small. This can often lead to people not only teasing you about diet or your funny-looking tan but can many times get people to question the amount of effort you put in to accomplish your goal. You may be challenged that you could be using your time more wisely, or possibly they may tell you that you're going overboard and don't need to invest so much time into your training. This is why I have always enjoyed a quote from EAS founder Bill Phillips: "Fanatic is a word the lazy use to describe the dedicated."

You see, if you are truly serious about getting into the type of shape that is presentable on stage before judges and a pretty large crowd, it's going to take sacrifice and lots of it. I've already discussed changing your diet, but that's just part of it. There are the countless hours in the gym; the giving up of certain ways of living to be sure you get adequate rest; the investment financially into supplements and all the quality food and gym memberships and-or home equipment; and the extra hours of cardio to lose that body fat that is in between your abs so you look sharp and chiseled. The motto of bodybuilding is ageless because it will always be true: *"No pain, no gain."*

There is true pain in resistance training. That's exactly what people who lift weights are doing—putting their muscles under a great deal of stress and pushing them to limits they can no longer endure. The weights provide a much greater resistance then the simple gravity we deal with every day. That resistance helps to tear down the muscle fibers, and with proper diet and rest, the fibers get built up again, both bigger and stronger. The more resistance you put your muscles under, the greater the payoff for all your training. Hard work, dedication, and sacrifice all go hand in hand, and the more resistance we get, the further we can go. It's like the old saying, "What does not kill you makes you stronger." Looking

70

good on stage is going to take sacrifice, and if you are going to achieve your goal, you are going to have to deny yourself and do whatever it takes to get the job done. That's not a fanatic; that's dedication, commitment, faithfulness, and passion manifested in the sculpting of the human body.

I cannot tell you how many times it would have seemed so much easier to just stay in bed in the morning or go hang out with the boys instead of going to the gym to get my workout in. You see, the first obstacle to overcome in the battle of discipline is your flesh.

>*The spirit is willing, but the body is weak.*
>*(Matt. 26:41)*

Jesus really hit the nail on the head with this one. There is always the air of excitement about getting to the gym, seeing friends, and getting a good pump going. But sometimes getting there is not always as exciting on a really cold morning or a beautiful evening after work. Sometimes you just want to relax. In your heart you want to train, but you start to make up excuses about why you deserve a break. I can remember them clearly because I still hear some of them in my head today.

1) What's the big deal if you miss just one workout?
2) Oh, those brownies won't make you fat
3) You worked hard today; you don't need to hit the weights.

It's almost like a tug-o-war starts to take place. To be honest, the battle starts in the mind. If you can't master this mind game, then you might as well say good-bye to your dreams. But if you can purpose to make it happen no matter what, then look out world! You must get to the gym, eat the right stuff, push out those extra, excruciatingly painful last couple of reps, and be disciplined enough to tell your body what it is going to do. If your mind is not in it, then your body will not follow. Sacrifice is something you decide in your heart before it takes place.

Many times before I actually joined a gym, I was thinking all day long about the workout I would have in my garage later in the evening. The only problem was that my gym was an outdoor garage, it was the middle of winter, and there was no heat with about six inches of snow on the ground. Trust me, there was a lot of battling going on in my head before I trekked out the back door and opened up that garage door to turn on the lights and see that *ice cold* steel.

Let me say this: the first few sets were very difficult. I was in layers of sweats. Even with gloves on, the barbell and dumbbells felt so cold it was painful. Yet even with these extreme conditions, something strange would always happen. About ten to fifteen minutes into it, the cold didn't seem so bad, the snow was more of a pleasure than a distraction, and the workout was getting very good. The sacrifice was always worth it. The post-workout celebration was that much tastier because I was willing to do whatever it took to get to my goal. I had a vision in my head of what I wanted to accomplish. I was going to endure hard training that I could not afford to skip out on no matter what the weather was like. I wanted to be able to compete on a stage against other bodybuilders. If that goal was going to become a reality, then the sacrifice had to be made.

I will never forget the time I was preparing for my first show back in 1990. I was a bit down on my luck and had rented my first apartment. Unfortunately, I could not afford my car payment and rent. Long story short, I returned the car and many years later had to pay a large fee to finish off the commitment I made with them. I was living close to Rosedale Queens, and my job was in Rockville Centre, about eight miles away. My only solution was to buy a bike.

My daily routine was to wake up about 5:00 a.m., have some breakfast, and hit the road by 6:00 a.m. I would put in an 8 hour work day and then ride my bike about two miles to Lynbrook where Gold's Gym was located. I'd work out for about an hour and then ride six miles home. If I wanted to eat, I had to ride my bike to work. If I wanted to train the right way for my first show,

I had to ride my bike to the gym six miles away. It was a sacrifice but one I was willing to make.

> *Everyone who competes in the games goes into strict training. They do it to get a crown that will not last; but we do it to get a crown that will last forever. Therefore I do not run like a man running aimlessly; I do not fight like a man beating the air. No, I beat my body and make it my slave so that after I have preached to others, I myself will not be disqualified for the prize. (1 Cor. 9:25–27)*

In recent years, as I have already mentioned, boxing has become quite a passion of mine. On May 16, 2009, I had my first amateur fight at world-renowned Gleason's Gym in Brooklyn, New York. Once my coach and I decided on that fight date, the heat got turned up. It was very clear to me that the training for a boxer was truly tougher than any fight he may have. When Coach said he was going to turn things up, he meant it. I was going to have to sacrifice many things to be ready for the fight. Knowing I had to weigh in at 168 pounds to be able to qualify for the chance to compete that night meant that my diet and cardio would have to be at their best. I would truly be pushed to the limit since that's a weight I have not been at in many moons.

Sometimes training took place at 6:30 a.m., and I was literally punching the crust out of my eyes. You know how hard it was to leave my family in their soft, comfy beds to go get punched in the head or do some drills that brought me close to losing my late-night protein shake almost every time. Other days it was running five miles and then shortly after, about an hour or so, I would do any combination of sparring, conditioning, bag work, or footwork. To say pre-fight training is tough would be an understatement, but just like stepping onstage, stepping in a ring would be foolish unless you truly knew in your heart you were as prepared as you could be. In fact, as I mentioned in chapter 5, I suffered my first loss that night, and while I was in the locker room getting changed, another boxer said these words to me, "You can play baseball, you can play football, you can play hockey, but you can't play boxing." I knew exactly what that meant the moment he said it.

Why do athletes do these things? Why do they make such great sacrifices? Why do they push themselves to places many would say is fanatical? I'll tell you why—it's because of the amazing benefits that come out of the hard work. You see, it's the benefits that come from all this sacrifice that keep you hungry. It's the knowledge that there are going to be big rewards for the effort that you are willing to put in while many others would rather flip on a TV and play with a remote.

The immediate benefits we see from being a bodybuilder or being in excellent condition are as follows. One benefit is that *you look good.* Almost all the people I know who got involved in the gym scene were there because they wanted to improve the way they looked in the mirror or improve the way they performed on the field. Appearance is an amazing benefit of resistance training. Arnold stated those words in *Pumping Iron* when he talked about how from every angle the way clothes fit a bodybuilder looks great. Mike O'Hearn, another famous bodybuilder once wrote an article about well-developed shoulders that really made sense. He talked about a man who would go out and spend a ton of money on an Armani suit. When he gets that suit home, he hangs it on a beautiful, big cedar hanger so it looks full and stately even when it's not being worn. He compared that suit being worn on a guy with poor shoulder development as hanging that same suit on a flimsy wire hanger; it just would not look right. He really got me training my delts hard after getting that visual in my mind.

At this stage of my life and my more modest way of dressing still does not negate the fact that having a muscular, symmetrical, and defined appearance makes you feel confident and good about yourself. It was not too long ago when I was bending down to pick up a pen from the floor and I felt blood rush to my head because the pants were so tight. I actually bent a bit sideways to relieve the pressure because my gut had grown so wide it was uncomfortable to even touch my toes, if I could. Glad that changed!

Another amazing benefit is *the health aspect*. When I started training for boxing, my cholesterol was about 260 according to the New York Blood Center, where I try to donate blood a couple of times a year. After nine months of tough boxing, weightlifting, and conditioning, I was notified by the NYBC that my cholesterol had dropped down to 198. I was so excited about that fact. I didn't actually start training like that to lower my cholesterol; it just turned out to be a benefit.

My training has not just made me look healthy on the outside but is truly changing my health from the inside out. As a lifelong sufferer of asthma, I have never used my inhaler *less* than I do now. Although I always keep my inhaler nearby just in case, it seems for me, the harder I work on pushing my lungs to deal with diminished oxygen from running, sprinting, sparring, squatting, etc., the less I need help breathing when I'm going about my daily activities and breathing at a normal rate. In the midst of all of this, *my ability to play with my kids* as long and as hard as I want is awesome. I have an eight-year-old and a ten-year-old. These girls are a gift from God. I feel so bad when parents just cannot engage in playing with or running around with their children because of their health.

Some athletes also have the benefit of *financial gain* from all their hard work. There is no need to really cover this topic as the media often reminds us of how much money many of the premier athletes make in sports today. Still, many compete at this type of level, be it novice or amateur, to win the prize. It could be a trophy or a title. It could be something as important as respect. All of these are plausible benefits of sacrifice.

Honestly, for me the greatest benefit is to *find out what I'm really made of.* You see, I feel that when you get to a place where you are no longer challenged, you are at a place where you have no purpose or reason for being. I know life is challenging enough. Marriage, children, career—they all take a lot of energy and time to be good at. I love Rick Warren's recent quote on Twitter about marriage, "Theprimary purpose of marriage is to make you holy, not happily everafter. Nothing challenges our self-centeredness more."

75

Marriage, parenting, work, etc., truly bring you to a point where you see what you are made of by how you handle the tough times and the valleys of life while trying to be the best you can at those areas. I also feel there is a place beyond that. For some it's sports, and for others it's something else, like people who have a dream birthed in them and they strive to climb the summit of Everest or sail across the Atlantic. When it comes to bodybuilding or boxing, I compete(d) against others on stage and in the ring, but the greatest foe I have is me. The greatest competition I face is the guy I look at in the mirror every morning. Whatever he is capable of now, whatever he has accomplished in the past, even though I am now forty-three, I want to do better. Every time I arrive at another goal, conquer another obstacle, fulfill another dream, it's time to push again.

Godliness:

There is no way I can start writing about this topic without pointing out the greatest sacrifice of all time: Jesus Christ! If we think about what He actually did for us, there is only one conclusion that can be drawn: Oh, how He loves us!

Let's take a minute and remember the sacrifice in totality. First, He left the beauties of heaven for a manger that animals would eat out of. Second, He left the worship of angels for the curses of men. Third, He left the throne of glory for the cross of Calvary. Do you realize how humiliating it was for Jesus to become one of us, one of His lowly creations? You might not think it's a big deal, but when You are the Creator of the universe and become equal to one of Your creations and then allow what You have created to torment and execute You, that's humiliating.

By the way, what about that execution? Talk about a sacrifice. The Bible gives vivid details in the Old Testament about specific animals that were to be used for sacrifices. When John the Baptist described Jesus as the Lamb of God, he was saying Jesus was going to take the place of an animal. Let's face it—He was surely treated as one. The beating He endured was relentless. He suffered in all facets: emotional (in the garden), physical (at the hands of all who beat him), and spiritual (when He was forsaken by the Father). Yet all of this was something He did willfully because He loved us so much. In fact, Jesus went as far as to state that He laid down His life and that nobody took it from Him.

> *The reason my Father loves me is that I lay down my life—only to take it up again. No one takes it from me, but I lay it down of my own accord. I have authority to lay it down and authority to take it up again. This command I received from my Father. (John 10:17–18)*

When I think of the way Jesus was willing to sacrifice Himself for me, I realize just how much I want to do for Him! I mean, let's face it—if I'm going to beat myself to get into shape so I might attain an earthly prize, how much more should I be willing to sacrifice my life for the rewards that Jesus has already attained for me through the cross?

Let me stress that this is all about wanting to do for Him. I don't have to! That would not be sacrifice; that would be personal gain! Let's recognize this truth. We cannot earn our salvation, as we already stated before. Jesus paid for us on the cross. My sacrifice is about honoring Him with my life as a sign of thanksgiving for all He has done for me!

> *Therefore, I urge you, brothers, in view of God's mercy, to offer your bodies as living sacrifices, holy and pleasing to God—this is your spiritual act of worship. (Rom. 12:1)*

Remember that living for Jesus is about attaining a crown that is greater than any trophy I could ever receive. In fact, that crown of salvation that Jesus purchased for me with His life is greater than any of the benefits I mentioned just a moment ago under physical training. And remember this passage, which is well worth repeating:

> *No, I beat my body and make it my slave **so that after I have preached to others, I myself** will not be disqualified for the prize. (1 Cor. 9:27)*

It was also the apostle Paul who said these words:

> *For our light and momentary troubles are achieving for us an eternal glory that far outweighs them all. (2 Cor. 4:17)*

What was light and momentary? He was shipwrecked, hungry, naked, cold, beaten, whipped, and stoned (with rocks!) for the gospel of Jesus. He did this with joy, as he wanted to offer his body as a living sacrifice for the God who gave his life for him. The Bible pictures for us a reward that will last forever, for eternity.

Just as mentioned in chapter 2, Paul, as well as all those who strive to live for Jesus, took the Lord's words to heart when he said:

> *If anyone would come after me, he must deny himself and take up his cross daily and follow me.*
> *(Luke 9:23)*

I have come to a firm conclusion in my short-lived life. If I am willing to give up so much and sacrifice to such extremes as bodybuilding and boxing demand, then dying to myself and living for my Savior is an absolute!

Before I go on, I must interject at this point with the concept of the resistance God sends to us during this lifetime. In His own words, Jesus told us in John 16:33, "In this world you will have trouble ..."

This trouble is what we often see as life's adversities. It may come at us in various ways: persecution for honoring God, sickness, financial distress, relational problems, etc. The problems we face in this world or the trouble that Jesus called it is a resistance of sorts very similar to the resistance of the weights used by a bodybuilder. Jesus wants to use these moments in life to get us to grow. We had a saying in Bible school, "You can get bitter or better!"

Honestly, if we never have a problem in life, then we will never get the chance to really see what we are made of. Unless someone rubs you the wrong way, how do you know if you can forgive? When you are hurt or face things in life that are difficult, you get to look at yourself with sober judgment, like looking into a mirror. These moments can make or break you. God wants to use these moments of resistance to make you stronger so you can be used to do more for His kingdom and be a greater blessing to others.

I read about the palm trees in Florida and how they bend a great deal during hurricane season, yet they do not break. The reason for this is that after each storm, their roots go deeper into the ground. Each moment of adversity for us should help us to get even deeper with our Lord. We should be more grounded and even stronger after a trial instead of getting mad at God or even worse, walking away from Him. Resistance in this life is not easy, but the sacrifice is well worth it. As I mentioned about negatives in chapter four under the Physical Training section, the negatives we experience will probably hurt really bad. They are non-stop pain. You can barely breathe as each repetitions success is built on the fact that you are exhausted and have no strength left to push or pull. It's in those negative times that our greatest results can be achieved. Negatives hurt so much that many choose not to utilize them and opt out on their benefits. In life we have many things that we see as negatives and indeed they may be just that but instead of seeing those moments as times when God did not care about us we should start understanding them for what they really are. Moments that God is using in our lives to help us grow in ways we may never have imagined. In fact, that adversity or resistance may be the answer to a prayer that you lifted up to God about becoming more like him.

Listen to Hebrews 12:7

> *Endure hardship as discipline; God is treating you*
> *as sons.*

Hardships are a form of discipline which this book is all about. People run from it and I myself do not jump for joy when hardship comes rather I choose to see each trail as another rep toward becoming who Christ wants me to be. I'll let those *negatives* become a way to get better instead of a weight that would crush me. Look at how the writer of Hebrews challenges us a few verses later:

> *Therefore, strengthen your feeble arms and weak*
> *knees (Hebrews 12:12)*

These hardships, trials and negatives of life are exactly what God will use to get us to grow. They are what strengthen us to raise our hands to praise God in the midst of adversity. They are what build us up to eventually hit our knees in prayer instead of bang our head against the wall in hopelessness. This of course is only going to happen when we choose to learn from what life throws at us:

> *No discipline seems pleasant at the time, but painful. Later on, however, it produces a harvest of righteousness and peace <u>for those who</u> <u>have been</u> <u>trained by it</u>. (Hebrews 12:11)*

The sacrifice Jesus is looking for is one of loyalty, commitment, faithfulness, etc. I am not talking about the sacrifice that was needed because of a sin that was committed. Animals were killed to cover the sins of man. The sacrifice I'm talking about is one of love and devotion to the Lord, not a sacrifice to cover my sin; Jesus did that for me.

Even the Lord himself reminded Israel:

> *To obey is better than sacrifice, and to heed is better than the fat of rams. (1 Sam. 15:22)*

No, God is looking for a sacrifice of holy living, or as the Psalmist wrote:

> *Let them give thanks to the Lord for his unfailing love and his wonderful deeds for men. Let them sacrifice thank offerings and tell of his works with songs of joy. (Ps. 107:21–22)*

This is a true believers' heartbeat. It's what drives them to see Christianity as the greatest journey mankind could experience. It's why the church is the greatest team ever assembled! We are loyal to our King. Our King laid His life down. I'm not a history buff, but I have yet to hear about a king who gave his life so his subjects could have peace. We usually hear about the king being hidden or moved to an undisclosed location during times of war so no harm would come his way. As a believer in Christ, I believe this is not my home, just as Jesus told Pilate that His kingdom was not of this world.

The benefits of sacrificial living for Christ are amazing. We can list each one just as we did for the "Physical Training" section. *First is the fact that leaving all for Jesus gives us the promise of reward:*

> **And everyone who has left houses or brothers or sisters or father or mother or children or fields for my sake will receive a** *hundred* **times as much and will inherit eternal life. (Matt. 19:29)**

> **Store up for yourselves treasures in heaven, where moth and** *rust* **do not destroy, and where thieves do not break in and steal. (Matt. 6:20)**

Not only are there eternal rewards, but there are beautiful benefits for the here and now as well.

I don't live my life for rewards from the Lord. Don't get me wrong: I always ask for health, protection, and prosperity for my family and me, but if I go through a valley, then so be it. I do, however, know that the Lord has promised me certain things in this world as a byproduct of honoring His Word in my life. He has told me that He is a rewarder of those who diligently seek Him. Sacrifice is a part of that diligence. It's very easy for people to give up their journey when things get tough,

> **To him who** *overcomes,* **I will give the right to eat from the tree of life, which is in the paradise of God. (Rev. 2:7)**

Second, you please the Lord! As Romans 12 stated, we learn God's good and pleasing will as we offer ourselves as living sacrifices. When we walk in His will, we will bring pleasure to the Lord. The Bible tells us:

> *Live as children of light … and find out what pleases*
> *the Lord. (Eph. 5:8, 10)*

If we can know what pleases the Lord, then it would make sense to do those things.

Third, we look like Christ. In the natural, our sacrifice achieves for us a look that is pleasing to the eye; spiritually our sacrifice achieves for us a look that is pleasing to the Lord. Remember that our representation of Jesus in this world may be the only Christ people get to see. We are even called ambassadors for Him. How amazing that we could have the look of the Son of God by how we honor Him with our living. This is truly attainable for those who are Spirit led, as the Word tells us:

> *His divine power has given us everything we need*
> *for life and godliness through our knowledge of him*
> *who called us by his own glory and goodness.*
> *(2 Peter 1:3)*

Fourth, sacrificial living is a sign of spiritual health. It's an indication that the things of God take precedence over all other things in your life. I think often about how many people who profess Christ are constantly wasting days, months, and years of their precious time here on earth. They are constantly getting into situations and struggling with sin instead of having victory over sin. Week after week, they are running to an altar for forgiveness for the same struggles. They become victims of the constant cycle of repentance instead of soaring like eagles and winning the lost for Christ. I thank Jesus for the forgiveness He has given me, even for the stuff I still do. Yet, there is a difference between tripping and being bound. Spiritually healthy people are actively involved in the war on souls. They are not constantly in the MASH unit trying to get healed again. They should be running the race with perseverance right until the end!

The fifth and final benefit I want focus on, although I'm sure you could identify more, is that you get to see what you're really made of! Just as previously mentioned, a life truly committed to Jesus will involve obedience to His Word. We are called to work out our salvation with fear and trembling. We are to look at the light of Scripture and allow it to guide our steps and direct our paths in life. Scripture goes against the grain of who we are when it comes to the desires of our human nature. We are naturally selfish, not selfless. Jesus showed us selflessness through His sacrifice. He did for us what we could not do for ourselves. He saved us from our sins!

As one of the board members of our church says it, "We all enter earth SDOA—spiritually dead on arrival. It is the zombie apocalypse, biologically alive yet spiritually dead." When you willingly lay down your life for the cause of Christ simply because He loved you first, you get to look at yourself with sober judgment. The greatest obstacle of serving Christ I have is me. No matter how bad Anthony wants to get in the way, I want to do more for my Jesus. I want to push further for my Lord. I don't want to live off yesterday's blessings; I want to make new testimonies for the kingdom of God. Sacrificial living has shown me that for sure:

> *You, dear children, are from God and have overcome them, because the one who is in you is greater than the one who is in the world. (1 John 4:4)*

Things to Ponder

1) Do you find yourself making excuses not to follow your goal (God), or do you have every reason in the world to do whatever it takes?

2) What are some of the battles you are wrestling with in your mind? Do you recognize how this battle will impact the next step you take?

3) Do you truly recognize how great of a sacrifice Christ made for you when He went to the cross?

4) Are you starting to find out what you are really made of?

CHAPTER 7

A "RESTED" DEVELOPMENT

By the seventh day God had finished the work he had been doing; so on the seventh day he rested from all his work. (Gen. 2:2)

Physical Training:

After all that hard training, sweating, and effort, you can be drained both physically and mentally. In the heat of competition, if things don't work out the way you had dreamed, you can even be drained emotionally. One of the best rewards I did not mention in our previous chapter is one that comes after every workout or contest. The shower! It's in there that you know the task is over, you get back to balance, and you get to start relaxing. I can't think of anything that feels as good as that nice, warm shower after a training session.

This moment of rest is really not the focus of this chapter. That's just a moment all athletes enjoy—or at least I hope you do. If not, please, for the sake of those who know you, take the *SHOWER*. What I really want to concentrate on is the idea of proper rest. You see, the intangibles of bodybuilding, such as diet and exercise, are surrounded by other important variables for you to get maximum results for all the hard work you put in. All the other areas I've mentioned are about doing. Rest is about not doing. It's about allowing that body to recover from the wages of war you have been putting it through.

When you get the bodybuilding bug or any other fire in your belly toward accomplishment, it's hard to hold back. I was so naïve when I began my journey toward getting on stage and competing. I was in the gym all the time. The amazing thing to me was not only did I find time to go to the gym, but I never really got bored of it. As a young guy who really did not have much in my heart for doing the things God wanted, I was out to discover what life was like. I thought I could party all night, work all day, and train like an animal without any adverse effects. I had heard about getting enough sleep and that there was a danger in overtraining, but I figured I was young and that must have been for the "older" guys.

Little did I know what eight hours of sleep could do for the body in regard to recovery and repairing all those muscle fibers I was tearing down in those grueling workouts. In my mind, I had no idea that you don't grow when you are lifting the weights but rather when you are at rest or sleeping. In regard to overtraining, I could not keep my hands off the weights. As often as I could be in the gym, and as many times a week as I could train a body part, I would. I eventually got into a two times a week for each body part routine, but I never really wanted to take off. I thought I was working harder than the other guys and showing discipline when in actuality, I was hurting myself and my chances of making faster gains.

I remember just before my first show, I was in the gym training some back and biceps, and someone who knew I was competing asked me what I was doing. I answered, "Getting in a last-minute workout." He just stared at me since the show was the next day and said, "You should be home resting." He understood that allowing my body to rest would not only help me recover but would allow my body to respond to the lack of water and salt depleting we were doing to get the skin tight. It would also help me be sharp and save all my energy for that tough pre-judging that was a day away.

I guess it was just hard for me to trust the fact that if I did not do anything, I would get better—that if I trusted my body's ability to heal and repair, I would actually make some strides. Trust me, a good night's sleep would have been welcomed, and getting things at home cleaned up or relaxing would not have been a bad idea either. It sounds so simple, but I just could not wrap my mind around the idea of doing nothing but allowing myself to have down time away from the gym. I would actually feel guilty, like I was doing something wrong if I didn't break a sweat or get my heart rate up. I felt like the only way to make any strides was to have an amazing pump and feel stiff and sore the next day.

Now that I'm older, I understand the benefits of rest. In fact, let's say I probably cannot be accused of not getting enough rest. During the training that I described for my first fight, my body started talking to me loud and clear. It was the Wednesday before the boxing event I was scheduled to be in that Saturday night. I was running five miles a day and had an hour of boxing training to follow. We cut back to three miles, which I did Monday through Wednesday. I saw my coach at the gym and just told him I was exhausted. His advice was just to relax till the big day, and that's exactly what I did. I got plenty of rest and had no need to do any shadow boxing or bag work. I just needed to stop.

The medical benefits of allowing your body to rest are without question. According to the Division of Sleep Medicine at Harvard Medical School, your body manages and requires sleep in much the same way that it regulates the need for eating, drinking, and breathing. Extensive research has been done on the effects of sleep. These studies have consistently shown that sleep plays a vital role in promoting physical health, longevity, and emotional well-being.[2] This explains why, after a good night's sleep, you feel better, your thoughts are clearer, and your emotions are less fragile. Without adequate sleep, judgment, mood, and ability to learn and retain information are weakened. In a study appearing in the July issue of *SLEEP*, Cheri Mah, a researcher in the Stanford Sleep Disorders Clinic and Research Laboratory, has shown that basketball players at the elite college level were able to improve their on-the-court performance by increasing their amount of total sleep time.[3] Mah also went on to do studies with other premier athletes and discovered similar results. Here are eleven benefits that were listed on Huffingtonpost.com in regards to proper rest:[4]

---

2   "Why Sleep Matters," Division of Sleep Medicine at Harvard Medical School. Accessed 2008 http://healthysleep.med.harvard.edu/healthy/matters

3   "Snooze you win? It's true for achieving hoop dreams, says study," MICHELLE L. BRANDT. Stanford School of Medicine. Accessed July 1, 2011 http://med. stanford.edu/ism/2011/july/sleep.html

4   "11 Surprising Health Benefits Of Sleep," the Huffington Post.com, Inc. part of AOL Lifestyle. Accessed 2013 http://www.huffingtonpost.com/2011/02/02/ sleep-health-benefits

Eleven Surprising Health Benefits of Sleep:

- Improve memory
- Live longer
- Curb inflammation
- Spur creativity
- Be a winner
- Improve your grades
- Sharpen attention
- Have a healthy weight
- Lower stress
- Avoid accidents
- Steer clear of depression

Godliness:

Being a Christian is not something you do when you're at church or when you're about to pray for your next meal. A committed believer is a follower of Christ twenty-four/seven, 365! So when I write about the spiritual evaluation of rest, please don't think we ever stop honoring Jesus with our lives. This rest I want to talk about and what the Bible describes is something that is much needed for anyone who plans on making a difference in the kingdom of God. Before we go there, let's break down what Jesus said:

> *Come to me, all you who are weary and burdened, and I will give you rest. (Matt. 11:28)*

Jesus is making it clear that the same world that is going to give us trouble is also going to eventually wear us out. It's at that point of weariness that the Devil does his best work. In those hours of restlessness, the Devil speaks his craftiest lies. He tells the wife whose husband cheated that drunkenness or drugs is the only way to deal with the pain. He deceives the young girl who wants to fit in that she should give in to peer pressure and give herself away before she's married. He blinds the mind of the man who is about to be arrested for embezzling people's retirements and makes him think suicide is the best way to handle the situation. After all, how could your family look at you again when they find out how you ripped off all those senior citizens from their life savings?

What Satan has to offer us is guilt and shame and regrets. What the Devil offers is a constant yearning that will never be satisfied. The pleasures of this world run dry, and they are designed to tear us down. Just look at the Ten Commandments. As you start to live in a way contrary to God's law, you start to live in stressed-out situations. Lying, stealing, disrespecting parents, etc., all lead to moments of stress, shame, and hurt. Sometimes it's simply all of the above.

In stark contrast, Jesus offers the exact opposite. He offers rest.

What an amazing place to find yourself, especially when you have come from the rat race of society, living to please everyone else but God. You were trying to get the things in your world in order. You were trying to keep the chaos at a minimum and in your own strength keep everything moving along smoothly. Then life just got too overwhelming. Emptiness was eating away at you despite success and financial wellness. How did things get this way? How did everything start to seem so out of order? You were doing everything you were taught. You were a good wife, a model student, and an exemplary employee. How did things get so messed up? It's because you have been trusting in yourself instead of putting your hope in the one who knows you better than you know yourself. Jesus is asking you in this passage, "Are you ready to have what you need?" He is the God who holds the worlds together. He keeps everything in order that   exists:

> *He is before all things, and in him all things hold*
> *together. (Col. 1:17)*

He now goes as far as to tell you that if your world is spinning out of control, if you're sick and tired of being sick and tired, He's got what you need. *Rest!* What a relief, and what a surprise. All that effort and searching, all that hard work and attention to detail, and Jesus says, "Don't do anything." He has exactly what we need and what we have been looking for. Psalm 23 says it   wonderfully:

> *The Lord is my shepherd, I shall not be in want.*
> *He makes me lie down in green pastures, he leads*
> *me beside quiet waters, he restores my soul. He*
> *guides me in paths of righteousness for his name's*
> *sake. Even though I walk through the valley of the*
> *shadow of death, I will fear no evil, for you are*
> *with me; your rod and your staff, they comfort me.*
> *You prepare a table before me in the presence of*
> *my enemies. You anoint my head with oil; my cup*
> *overflows. Surely goodness and love will follow me*

> *all the days of my life, and I will dwell in the house*
> *of the Lord forever.*

The rest we find in Him is our identity, our purpose, the "why we are here" of life. Everyone's expectations of who we should be melt away when we find out what He thinks of us. What a relief when we find out that He wants to carry the weight of our problems. After all, He carried the sins of the world, so our problems are pretty light for His shoulders.

> *Take my yoke upon you and learn from me, for I am*
> *gentle and humble in heart, and you will find rest*
> *for your souls. For my yoke is easy and my burden*
> *is light. (Matt. 11:29–30)*

Thank You, Jesus, for accepting me, not because of the works I have done but based on what You have done for me on the cross.

Now don't mistake serving the Lord from resting in Him. As we discussed already, faith without works is death. This is not about service; this is about surrender. It is about admitting my utter dependence on a God who is more than willing to give me all I need to not only make it in this world but to be a difference maker.

Rest also provides for us just what we need as soldiers in the army of God. I tell all of the members of our church that I would not ask of them to make more than two services a week. If they choose to do more than that, it's up to them, but I know that even in serving the Lord, we can tend to get fatigued or even burn ourselves out. There have been several times when I have told people they could not participate in another ministry because they are just stretching themselves too much.

As a pastor, it's my job to make sure the sheep stay healthy. As a Christian, I know the benefits of getting rest. My advice to one person was instead of being good at a lot of things, why not rest a little and be great at one or two things? The shame of this topic is that some very well-meaning individuals (just saying that to be nice) have made some people believe that if they are not in church every time the doors are open, they are in sin. I know of one young man who was volunteering at another church for almost seven hours a night several nights a week. You can't imagine how happy his wife was when I told him, "That's not going to happen with us." Many families are falling apart because we are busy caring about everyone else but forgetting about those who live under our roofs.

There is indeed a great benefit to rest, just like the growth gains that come to the human body at night when proper rest is acquired. The Bible says it this way:

> *The Lord is the everlasting God, the Creator of the ends of the earth. He will not grow tired or weary, and his understanding no one can fathom. He gives strength to the weary and increases the power of the weak. Even youths grow tired and weary, and young men stumble and fall; but those who hope in the Lord will renew their strength. They will soar on wings like eagles; they will run and not grow weary, they will walk and not be faint. (Isa. 40:28–31)*

Waiting on the Lord means we have admitted He is in control, and we know He has what we need to keep moving forward. Waiting on the Lord means we do not kick open doors for opportunity but rather let Him open them for us as He guides us in all things and in His time. As the passage goes on, it tells us that what we do in this spiritual truth will affect us in the natural. *We will mount up with wings like eagles.* Resting in the Lord will give us a better perspective of our current situation. We will see things from higher ground. We get a bird's-eye view of what God is up to. Think about it. When we rush to conclusions, when we jump the gun based on information we just heard, we tend to make rash decisions that can often leave us angry or hurting someone for no reason. That's why these biblical words hold such good advice:

> *Everyone should be quick to listen, slow to speak*
> *and slow to become angry. (James 1:19)*

When our strength is renewed (which we get when we rest in the Lord), we can let the Holy Spirit show us something or teach us a lesson in the middle of the ordeal, trial, or difficult time. The eagle is known to be powerful enough to fly up into the eye of the storm where there is peace, even in the midst of all the devastation that is going on around him. This restful view will only come when we give the Lord a chance to reveal His view on things.

That we will run and not grow weary is great news for all those who are growing tired. The more we rest in our Lord (remember, resting is what we are doing when we wait), the stronger we get. When simple adversity used to bring us to our knees in defeat, we now can hurdle obstacles of life in a single bound. The time we took to rest in Christ instead of trying to take control of the situation has now enabled us to do more than we could have ever done on our own.

We will walk and not faint. Even at the most difficult moments life can throw at us, we will still be moving forward for the cause of Christ. The enemy has a goal—to get you to retreat—and in order to make that happen, he must get you to stand still. He wants to stop all momentum that might lead you to the cross. Psalm 1 and Isaiah 40 are amazing illustrations of what happens to those who rely on their own strength instead of spending time mediating, waiting on, or resting in the Lord.

Let me compare them for you:

> *But those who hope in the Lord will renew their*
> *strength. They will soar on wings like eagles; they*
> *will run and not grow weary, they will walk and not*
> *be faint. (Isa. 40:31)*

Soar, run, walk—the person who waits never stops moving. At his very worst, he is walking!

Blessed is the man who does not walk in the counsel of the wicked or stand in the way of sinners or sit in the seat of mockers. (Ps. 1:1)

Walk, stand, sit—people who listen to the enemy will have their walks come to a screeching halt, and any momentum they had that was propelling them to the cross will become a distant memory as they plant themselves in a seat of deception. If they would have rested or waited on the Lord, they could have been renewed. Now their so-called walk has turned into a seat of hypocrisy and rebellion.

Things to Ponder

1) Can you tell when you are getting close to burning out? How does it affect you and your family?

2) Does God have control of your life, or do you? If you have control, then how have things been working out for you so far?

3) Does it bring you relief to know Jesus wants to carry the weight of your problems?

4) God wants us to move forward with Him; in what direction is your life headed?

5) Why is it so hard for us to just make time for God, both personally and with the church?

CHAPTER 8
THE CHANGE—UP

Physical Training:

You may have seen it on TV. You know the infomercials I'm talking about—P90X or the Insanity workouts. We see those pictures of the guy who, in ninety days, transformed his body from couch potato to muscle beach hunk or the lady who went from sitting at her desk eating Krispy Kreme to running in a triathlon.

What's the secret to these success stories? The secret is that there is no secret. These are two programs that really work. Why, you ask? They work because you actually have to break a sweat and push yourself. You don't strap on the magic belt to reduce your waist size or rub on the ancient crème to melt away the pounds. You actually have to be active and get your heart rate up, exert some energy, and push yourself to places you would normally never go.

The other key to these DVDs of fitness is the way they keep the body from being able to adjust to the workouts. The science behind it is that you constantly throw new exercises and movements at your body to keep your body in a place where it just did not see that coming. They use constant change to keep the body from being able to adapt or build a resistance to the training. This constant change puts our muscles in a place of surprise and in turn forces them to be used to their maximum capacity. It's like that when you have not trained for a while and you finally make it back to the gym. Even if you do some simple movements for arms, back, etc., you will most likely be pretty sore the next day. Keep doing that same routine over and over, and soon you will notice that getting sore is a thing of the past and you are just going through the motions.

Back in the day, well before the DVD and Tony Little (just had to mention him) and personal trainers on our TV sets, I trained with this constant change style of workout. It was actually called the High-Intensity Workout by Mike Metzer. Mike and his brother, Ray, were huge in the bodybuilding world when I got bit by the muscle bug. The idea was simple but grueling. You would plan to work out for about thirty minutes. You would get the gym set up with the weight you needed. You had a series of different exercises that would wind up targeting your entire body.

The kicker was that there was really no rest between sets. This was very tough to accept for a guy who wanted to tell everyone how much he benched during last night's workout. There was no way you could lift heavy on the bench press when you just did as many push-ups as you could until you dropped and then, without rest, got on the bench and maxed out. Body part after body part, you would attack. Set after set, you would grimace, spit, take deep breaths, and wish it was over. That was the first five minutes. The effort it took to complete this workout was a lot more than your usual session in the gym, and the reason was this: it did not allow room for complacency. There was no five-minute rest between sets. One after the other, the exercises came. Arms, back, chest, traps, and the most grueling part, legs!

I remember asking my now brother-in-law if he would like for me to give him a training session. Because he showed up to train and not play games, he gave it his all. It was not long before I had the privilege of finding out what he had eaten for dinner that evening. Yet, with the heart of a champ, he jumped right back in as soon as he was done "catching his breath." It wasn't pretty.

Unfortunately, we are creatures of habit, and once we get used to a routine, we tend to gravitate toward it because it's simply what we know. Ask any bodybuilder who knows what he is doing and he will let you know how important it is to do different movements to properly break down the muscles you want to grow and sculpt. When I work out, I always want to try to do a different type of workout from the last time I trained that body part. I may reuse an exercise that I did a few days before, but I want to always incorporate a new angle or position to the movement if I can. I'll try to mix it up with a different grip or some crazy high-rep to low-rep scheme. With all the new equipment in gyms today, there should be no problem coming up with creative workouts that will constantly keep your body in a state of shock and allow you to keep the gains coming at a constant pace. Change is good and in fact a must if you want to reach the level you desire and maximize all the hard work and see it birth true results.

Another thing that change brings us is a chance to experience something different. I know, as I stated, that many people are creatures of habit. We get into our routines and don't like anyone rocking our boat. They like the same food, the same TV shows, the same clothes, etc. You get what I mean; they just don't like change. The problem with this again is that you can very easily get stuck in a rut or what the bodybuilding world would call a plateau. You just don't make gains anymore no matter how hard you try. That's why changes are so important. It spices things up.

Look, I love chicken cutlet parm, but I don't want to eat it all the time. That would get boring, and eventually I would get sick of it. Changing up the meals is exciting. Eating something you never had before is fun and can make for some very enlightening and funny moments! Change adds that element of making things different and creating new challenges for your body to respond to—like when you add a new exercise or give up the weights that day for plyometrics. Maybe instead of heavy lifting you're going for max reps and negatives. Instead of loads of bag work or jump rope, you run a few miles and do some swimming.

They say variety is the spice of life; it is no different when it comes to training and wanting to truly make some serious gains. Isn't the whole idea behind our training to get us from where we are to where we want to be? As a bodybuilder, your goal is to change (improve) the way your body looks. A boxer wants to change (improve) his conditioning, footwork, hand skills, etc. In fact, any area of fitness or sports is a direct challenge to see how much change (improvement) you can make. If you're going to truly grow, then you're going to have to change.

Godliness

Immutable. That's a big word. It's a word that describes one of the incommunicable attributes of God. These are the things we will only be able to see in God Himself, such as divine, sovereign, etc. The word itself tells us that God does not change. Several Scriptures remind us of this truth.

I the LORD do not change. (Mal. 3:6)

Jesus Christ is the same yesterday and today and forever. (Heb. 13:8)

This is something we need to be very grateful for. He has made Himself known through His Word and has promised that He is not a man that He should lie. He will do what He said He will do. God has been consistent with this throughout the centuries. His Word has continually shown His greatness and mercy come to pass generation after generation, and we should all rejoice over it. We should be tremendously thankful that the Lord does not say, "You know what? Forget that forgiveness thing; you just don't deserve it."

Yet, in stark contrast to the fact that God does not change, we desperately need to. There are various ways the Lord brings change into our lives, and each way helps us on our journey to become more like Christ.

First there is a change in our ability to stand before the Lord. The Bible is clear that sinful man is in dire straits. He needs to be rescued from the consequences of sin. We have already covered much of this first point earlier in this book. To sum it up one more time, sin has entered into this world and separated the Creator (God) from His creation (us). There was and still is nothing we can do to get ourselves back in good standing with God, so Jesus came as the answer to the disease of sin. A dead person cannot resurrect him or herself; this takes the act of a sovereign, all-powerful God. Remember:

> *God made him who had no sin to be sin for us, so that in him we might become the righteousness of God. (2 Cor. 5:21)*

This sacrifice of God's only begotten Son changes those who accept His truth. Only through Christ can a person be saved. Listen to what the Bible says about the nature of a person who surrenders to the lordship of Christ:

> *Praise be to the God and Father of our Lord Jesus Christ! In his great mercy he has given us new birth into a living hope through the resurrection of Jesus Christ from the dead. (1 Peter 1:3)*

> *For you were once darkness, but now you are light in the Lord. Live as children of light. (Eph. 5:8)*

> *Therefore, if anyone is in Christ, the new creation has come: The old has gone, the new is here! (2 Cor. 5:17)*

Look at those words that are used. *New birth, your light, new creation,* and let's not forget:

> *Jesus replied, "Very truly I tell you, no one can see the kingdom of God unless they are born again."(John 3:3)*

These words tell us of a change in our standing before the Lord. The words that describe this transformation are justification and regeneration. Both of these words take place the moment we surrender to Christ as Savior

- Justification: We are in right standing with God.
- Regeneration: Our nature, our position in God's eyes has changed (from enemy of God to child of God).

104

This change was seen when Zacchaeus came into contact with Jesus:

> *Jesus entered Jericho and was passing through. A man was there by the name of Zacchaeus; he was a chief tax collector and was wealthy. He wanted to see who Jesus was, but because he was short he could not see over the crowd. So he ran ahead and climbed a sycamore-fig tree to see him, since Jesus was coming that way. When Jesus reached the spot, he looked up and said to him, "Zacchaeus, come down immediately. I must stay at your house today." So he came down at once and welcomed him gladly. All the people saw this and began to mutter, "He has gone to be the guest of a sinner." But Zacchaeus stood up and said to the Lord, "Look, Lord! Here and now I give half of my possessions to the poor, and if I have cheated anybody out of anything, I will pay back four times the amount." Jesus said to him, "Today salvation has come to this house, because this man, too, is a son of Abraham. For the Son of Man came to seek and to save the lost." (Luke 19:1–10)*

What a beautiful story of how having an encounter with the Son of God can change our standing from enemy (sinner) to son (child of God). The people did not get it, and they accused Jesus of being around a sinner, like it was something bad, but remember, that is why He came. He came for the Zacchaeuses and the Anthonys of this world, and He came for us even when we did not look so good.

> *But God demonstrates his own love for us in this: While we were still sinners, Christ died for us. (Rom. 5:8)*

How glad I am that this first point takes place—that Jesus wants to change us even if we don't look like we belong or act like we belong. Think about it—when the Lord was on the cross, He cried out, "Father, forgive them, for they know not what they do." He cried that out when no one was asking for forgiveness, no one deserved forgiveness, and He certainly didn't owe them forgiveness. Yet He wanted to give it. He wanted to change their standing. Even though people may not get it, I'm so glad Jesus got me!

Second, there is a change in our ability to serve the Lord.

> **The Spirit of the LORD will come powerfully upon you, and you will prophesy with them; and** *you will be changed into a different person.* **(1 Sam. 10:6)**

> *But you will receive power* **when the Holy Spirit comes on you;** *and you will be my witnesses* **in Jerusalem, and in all Judea and Samaria, and to the ends of the earth.** *(Acts 1:8)*

God's plan for us is not just for us to make it to heaven. His desire is not for us to simply say, "Thank You for the forgiveness. Now I'll sit in my comfy little world and wait for You to return." He has placed us in this world for a purpose. We are not to just hear the Word but do it. Doing His Word means that we are to be actively involved in what His kingdom is all about. The primary reason Jesus came to this world was to win the lost—to lead people to salvation from their sins. He calls us the body of Christ, as this book is partly titled. We are to be His hands, feet, mouth, etc., to as many people as possible.

This does not come easy. In fact, most people cringe at the idea of trying to tell someone their testimony or God's love for them. We often shy away because we don't want to be rejected or made to feel like a bother. Now I just need to say that the message we carry is so dynamic and vital for everyone, including those who don't know it, that their reaction should be secondary in light of the disease that is eating away at them. So God has provided a way for us to be able to step out of most of our comfort zones and find the strength to do the things He is asking us to do. We receive all we need to be frontline Christians by having God fill us with His Spirit. This is what both the Old and New Testaments are referring to when we read the two passages above.

We are changed into different people. You will receive power! Wow, what promises. God is getting a hold of us from the inside out and changing us into people we may have never thought we could become.

For me there can be no greater illustration than the apostle Paul. He was changed from trying to destroy the church to becoming one of the greatest pillars of the church. He wanted to abolish the name of Jesus at all costs, and he thought he was doing God a favor. He was convinced he was right. Then one day he met with God on the Damascus road, and that's where God changed his standing:

> *Meanwhile, Saul was still breathing out murderous threats against the Lord's disciples. He went to the high priest and asked him for letters to the synagogues in Damascus, so that if he found any there who belonged to the Way, whether men or women, he might take them as prisoners to Jerusalem. As he neared Damascus on his journey, suddenly a light from heaven flashed around him. He fell to the ground and heard a voice say to him, "Saul, Saul, why do you persecute me?" "Who are you, Lord?" Saul asked. "I am Jesus, whom you are persecuting," he replied. "Now get up and go into the city, and you will be told what you must do." (Acts 9:1–6)*

It's amazing how the guy who claimed to represent God did not even know who God was when he met Him face to face. After God changed Saul's position in heaven, He changed his ability to be used for God in the right way:

In Damascus there was a disciple named Ananias. The Lord called to him in a vision, "Ananias!" "Yes, Lord," he answered. The Lord told him, "Go to the house of Judas on Straight Street and ask for a man from Tarsus named Saul, for he is praying. In a vision he has seen a man named Ananias come and place his hands on him to restore his sight." "Lord," Ananias answered, "I have heard many reports about this man and all the harm he has done to your holy people in Jerusalem. And he has come here with authority from the chief priests to arrest all who call on your name." But the Lord said to Ananias, "Go! This man is my chosen instrument to proclaim my name to the Gentiles and their kings and to the people of Israel. I will show him how much he must suffer for my name." Then Ananias went to the house and entered it. Placing his hands on Saul, he said, "Brother Saul, the Lord—Jesus, who appeared to you on the road as you were coming here—has sent me so that you may see again and be filled with the Holy Spirit." Immediately, something like scales fell from Saul's eyes, and he could see again. (Acts 9:10–18)

Another amazing thing we can take note of is that when God fills you with His Holy Spirit, you can start to see things the way you're supposed to. Paul saw Jesus as a threat, but now he saw Him as the only hope. Paul was physically blind, but now, after his encounter with God, he could truly see. And it was not long before this change took him to a new place:

At once he began to preach in the synagogues that Jesus is the Son of God. All those who heard him were astonished and asked, "Isn't he the man who raised havoc in Jerusalem among those who call on this name?" (Acts 9:20–21)

They would not have believed the change unless they had seen it with their own eyes.

Third, there is a change in our ability to fully surrender to the Lord. As previously stated, our goal is to be perfect as our heavenly father is perfect (Matt. 5:48). In many prayer circles and intimate times with God, committed followers of Christ have asked God to bring this change within them. Very often the answer to this prayer is more than what we bargained for because if the God who does not change used suffering to build up His Son, then in order for us to change, suffering most likely will come:

> *During the days of Jesus' life on earth, he offered up prayers and petitions with fervent cries and tears to the one who could save him from death, and he was heard because of his reverent submission. Son though he was, he learned obedience from what he suffered and, once made perfect, he became the source of eternal salvation for all who obey him. (Heb. 5:7–9)*

Jesus learned obedience, and that means He had to endure all the suffering that came His way to pay the price for our sins. He had never felt pain like that before, in as many ways as it was inflicted upon Him. He had to face it all in His humanity so all of us could share in His redemption. Remember, He became a priest who could empathize with us in every way so that when we are faced with trials and valleys, we can recall His obedience and find the strength we need in the struggle.

God allows change to come into our lives. Sometimes it's good and sometimes it's really difficult, but change is going to come. The Father wants to build the character of His Son in us, and change is how He gets that character developed. If you're one of those people who say, "I'm not good with change," then you should probably hold on tight, as that's exactly the tool Christ is going to use to develop you into His child. Being like Jesus is exactly what our Father God wants:

> *For those God foreknew he also predestined to be*
> *conformed to the image of his Son, that he might be the*
> *firstborn among many brothers. (Rom. 8:29)*

Think of James's words:

> *Consider it pure joy, my brothers and sisters,*
> *whenever you face trials of many kinds, because*
> *you know that the testing of your faith produces*
> *perseverance. Let perseverance finish its work so*
> *that you may be mature and complete, not lacking*
> *anything. (James 1:2–4)*

I don't know what kind of resistance training God is going to bring your way spiritually. I do know that He is looking for a fully surrendered vessel to pour Himself into, and for us to be that mature sons or daughters of the Lord, God is going to change things up. Listen to Job's words as he dealt with all the changes he went through:

> *Your hands shaped me and made me. Will you now*
> *turn and destroy me? Remember that you molded*
> *me like clay. Will you now turn me to dust again?*
> *(Job 10:8–9)*

But what was the end result of his ordeals?

> *My ears had heard of you but now my eyes have*
> *seen you. Therefore I despise myself and repent in*
> *dust and ashes. (Job 42:5–6)*

He saw that although he went through great suffering and trials, God was still molding him in his later years. Although God praised Job in the first chapter of the book, he still had much more work to be done in him, more molding to take place. Change brings this process, and when you're committed to Christ to become more like Him, you recognize these moments are times to grow, not times to gripe. Since David had so much experience in both the good and bad situations of life and still trusted his God, he was able to pen these words:

> *Even though I walk through the darkest valley, I will fear no evil, for you are with me. (Ps. 23:4)*

Change taught him how to not fear but rather trust. Have full confidence that no matter what you are going through, the Lord has your best interest in mind. If you're going to truly grow, then you're going to have to change!

Anthony L. Pelella

Things to Ponder

1) What changes or new challenges are you willing to endure to see the growth you desire?

2) Have you ever been stuck in a rut or hit a plateau? How did you get out of it?

3) If God evaluated you spiritually right now, how would you look? Be sure this answer is according to the Bible and not your own opinion.

4) Can you think of a time in your life or in the life of someone you know when change that was thought to be scary turned out to be the best thing that could have happened?

CONCLUSION: THE SPIRIT OF THE RADIO

If you choose not to decide, you still have made a choice.
—RUSH

I have seen all the things that are done under the sun; all of them are meaningless, a chasing after the wind. (Eccles. 1:14)

Physical Training:

It was the early eighties, and there I was. I don't know how it happened, but I was there. Somehow, some way, my dad agreed to let me go to my first concert. It was my favorite rock group, Rush. I was standing in the Nassau Coliseum late at night with some of my buddies from Brentwood. My best friend's mom had picked us up and dropped us off at this amazing moment of my teenage years.

The people in the parking lot were countless, and the journey to get our tickets torn to see this band we had never heard live seemed to take forever. Finally, we got in. As we were walking around trying to desperately find our way through the giant coliseum, we heard it. What was it we heard, you ask? The sound that, even as I write these words, causes a huge smile to cover my face and laughter to fill my heart. It was Alex Lifeson playing a guitar riff from Rush's opening song called "The Spirit of the Radio."

At the second we heard the music start, my friends and I made a mad dash to find our section. There we were, running through what seemed to be an endless sea of people and a never-ending search for our seats. It turned out we were not too far away from our seats but had gone the wrong direction and pretty much ran around the entire auditorium before entering through the doorway that was right next to us when we started. As we entered the gateway to our section of seats, we looked out to see a floor covered with hands raised and people singing. As we gazed upon the sections filled with fans, all singing this anthem of joy, I was in awe. Although the band looked like they were two inches tall because I was so far away, I didn't care. I was there. It was live. And they sounded awesome.

Almost as soon as we got this Kodak memory lodged in our hearts, we started to hear something else—other people yelling, "Sit down! Get out of the way." We needed to find our seats and do it quickly. Finally we were seated, and I was ready to take it all in. We were listening to the music, and then my pal got a brilliant idea. "Let's try to find closer seats," he said.

Now, I'm not the type of guy who likes to take a risk like that. If it's a baseball game, concert, movie, whatever, I feel like I'm going to sit in the seats I paid for, and unless everyone leaves, I'm not taking a chance of bribing an usher or getting yelled at by other fans who know you're cheating your way in.

Besides that, that journey to find these new illegal seats was going to take time away from the show I had come to enjoy. Even though Rush looked like three guys who could fit on top of a trophy, I was content and did not want to miss a second of the show. I wanted to sing every word, clap my hands, and stomp my feet. Searching for unknown and uncertain seats meant that I would have to give up my current position and miss out. Even if the seats were better, it would be at the expense of missing some of the show, and I was not up for that.

Everything had come together. Dad said yes, we got the tickets before they sold out, I got the concert jersey, and I was sitting watching a live show. No, I was not going to miss a minute of this. Every second I had was going to be spent taking the whole experience in and not wasting it trying to find better seats. In fact, I wouldn't buy a drink, go to the bathroom, or look for a better deal on concert shirts. I was there to look, hear, and feel the music firsthand, and I did. I ran after I heard "The Spirit of the Radio," and when I finally captured access to it and all the songs that followed it, I was not letting go.

Godliness:

In my years of experience, I find one thing to be true in life. I always wanted to find things that would make me happy. I yearned for something that would bring me pleasure, joy, satisfaction. There were many different avenues to try to accomplish this task. I tried to make money, I tried to be popular, I tried drinking and partying, etc. I always felt good when meeting new ladies and thought that was the answer to most of my emptiness. Even bodybuilding for me was an attempt to fulfill a need inside of me, a need that never seemed to be met, no matter how hard I pursued the things I've mentioned.

After years of living and knowing what it's like to have Jesus in my life and also to be living without Him, I've learned a very valuable lesson. The things I mentioned are momentary. In other words, they are things you have to continually run after in order to keep the feeling alive. You may get a moment of pleasure or happiness, but the pleasure or joy is short lived, and then it's back to that empty feeling again, only to find yourself back on the hunt to try and satisfy that empty feeling again through some other method. It's kind of like what the band Loverboy talked about when they sang, "Everybody's working for the weekend." In stark comparison to those things I've already mentioned is the one thing in life I've found that is worth running after—my relationship with the one who gave His life for me: **Jesus**!

You see, Jesus is what I have been looking for all my life. In fact, He's what all people have been looking for, whether they recognize it or not. Either way, He truly is the one who fills the void in our hearts, and He does this in a way that can never be accomplished by anything else. We are all dead spiritually, and the only way for us to experience life is to come to a place where we become united to the author of life, the creator of our souls, the author of our faith. As the Bible says:

> *This day I call heaven and earth as witnesses*
> *against you that I have set before you life and death,*

116

*blessings and curses. Now choose life, **so that you and your children may live and that you may love the LORD your God, listen to his voice, and hold fast to him. For the LORD is your life. (Deut. 10:19–20a)***

Jesus is life. You don't really know what living is until you live for Jesus. We also need to remember the immortal words of Rush, my favorite rock band of my teenage years, in their song "Freewill." "If you choose not to decide, you still have made a choice."

For years I chased after cars, wine, and women. I even ran after "The Spirit of the Radio." Today I have learned that there is nothing like running after the Spirit of the Lord. And trust me, like my friend trying to get me out of my seat in the show and maybe miss what was happening, there is an enemy who is trying to continually get me to try something else and miss what God has planned for me in this life.

As steadfast as I was about watching that show, I'm just as steadfast today about standing with the Lord. I don't want to miss a second of what God is doing or how He is touching people's lives. The ultimate sense of accomplishment is not based on chasing the things of this world but rather being called a child of God. Of all the titles God has blessed me with—*son, husband, daddy*—none of them compare with the title *child of God*. What the world has to offer is quickly fleeting and leads to destruction. What God has to offer is never ending and leads to eternal life. I guess it can be summed up by the man who had it all in life and knows the pleasures of both the flesh and the Lord.

Now all has been heard; here is the conclusion of the matter: Fear God and keep his commandments, for this is the whole duty of man. (Eccles. 12:13)

Game Over!

WWW.THEBODYBUILDERBOOK.COM

Made in the USA
Charleston, SC
09 December 2016